the
SECRET LIFE
of a
SUBMISSIVE

A True Story

SARAH K

HARPER

This book is a work of non-fiction based on the author's experiences.
In order to protect privacy, names, identifying characteristics, dialogue,
location and details have been changed or reconstructed.

HARPER

An imprint of HarperCollins*Publishers*
77–85 Fulham Palace Road,
Hammersmith, London W6 8JB

www.harpercollins.co.uk

First published by Harper 2012

1 3 5 7 9 10 8 6 4 2

© Sarah K 2012

Sarah K asserts the moral right to
be identified as the author of this work

A catalogue record for this book is
available from the British Library

ISBN: 978-0-00-750621-7

Printed and bound in Great Britain by
Clays Ltd, St Ives plc

MIX
Paper from
responsible sources
FSC **FSC C007454**
www.fsc.org

FSC™ is a non-profit international organisation established to promote
the responsible management of the world's forests. Products carrying the
FSC label are independently certified to assure consumers that they come
from forests that are managed to meet the social, economic and
ecological needs of present and future generations,
and other controlled sources.

Find out more about HarperCollins and the environment at
www.harpercollins.co.uk/green

the SECRET LIFE *of a* SUBMISSIVE

To P – I have never felt so loved.

Chapter One

'I know nothing about sex
because I was always married.'
Zsa Zsa Gabor

'So if you could do *anything*, anything at all, what would you do?' I asked, handing round the after-dinner mints.

Across the table, Gabbie, who is one of my oldest and best friends, and who was busy helping herself to the last slice of cheesecake, said, 'I'm assuming we're not talking about hang-gliding here, are we?'

'No. In bed.'

'In bed?' said Helen. 'That restricts it a bit. How about *out* of bed?'

'You know what I mean: if you could do anything *sexually*.'

'Oh, you're way too coy to be a pornographer,' snorted Gabbie.

'Do the things we've already done count?' asked Joan.

We all turned to look at her. Joan is small, lovely, and looks like butter wouldn't melt. Back in the mists of time she'd been a tour rep for Thomson's and up until now what had happened on tour had most definitely stayed on tour.

'Anything,' I repeated. 'Any time, any place, anywhere.'

'And then you're going to write about it?' said Helen, topping up her wine glass.

'Well, yes, if it's any good I will. I won't use any of your names, obviously, and I'll change it enough so that no one knows it was you.'

'That's a shame,' said Joan, taking another mint from the box. 'I'm sure Miguel and Antonio would be chuffed to bits to see their names up in lights.'

Everyone laughed. 'You're winding us up,' said Gabbie.

Joan pulled a face and then laughed. 'Oh, come on,' she said. 'We all did crazy things when we were younger.'

'I didn't,' I said, and this time it was me they all looked at. 'Well, it's true. I didn't. I was married by the time I was twenty.'

'Before then,' said Gabbie, 'you must have played around a bit.'

'I had a couple of boyfriends, but not that many. And Ray and I met when I'd just finished sixth form …' I began. 'You know that.'

Although I didn't say anything, in all the years we'd been together Ray had always preferred his sex the same way he enjoyed his food: plain, nothing fancy and without any peculiar ingredients. For him the very thought of anything that didn't involve fumbling around under the duvet with the lights off was a sign of moral turpitude, and if he had ever enjoyed it before, it wasn't the kind of thing you inflicted on your wife.

'Oh, that is classic,' snorted Helen. 'You're the one who is supposed to be writing a dirty book and you're the only one who's stuck to the straight and narrow. Fabulous.'

'It's not dirty, it's erotica, and this is exactly why I've got you lot over. So what would you do?'

We were having a fajita evening in the kitchen at Gabbie's cottage near Somerleyton.

We've been doing it for years. We used to meet up once a month when the children were smaller, but these days we get together when we can fit it into our increasingly busy lives. Every time we do it I wish we did it more.

We met at pre-natal classes in a scout hut in a little village just outside Cambridge. We've supported each other through backache, heartburn, teething, sleepless nights, terrible twos, troublesome teenagers, empty nests, dodgy marriages, cheating husbands and messy divorces. We've wept with each other, laughed with each other, got drunk with each other, and helped each other move house and move on. Remarkably we're all still friends.

Spread out over Gabbie's huge farmhouse kitchen was the debris of wrap-them-up-yourself chicken fajitas, tortilla chips, sour cream, salsa, potato wedges, white wine, Spanish beer and a big jug of margarita mix. We'd eaten our way through assorted tubs of Ben & Jerry's and a twice-baked New York cheesecake made by Joan who, after years of abstinence on the kitchen front, had started working in a cookshop, taken up the apron and turned out to be the most amazing cook.

Gabbie is a solicitor, well spoken, tall and skinny, with the most fabulous long, straight, brown hair. Whatever she's doing, she always looks as if she has just been ironed.

Helen is a gardener: strawberry blonde, ruddy complexion, capable, funny, always wears trousers or shorts and smiles a lot. There's Joan, tiny, pretty, dark-haired Joan, who manages a shop and is a deacon at her local church. And then there's me, Sarah, and I'm a writer.

I'd been writing romantic fiction for the best part of twenty years, creating modern fairy tales about handsome, flawed, lovable heroes and complex women with complicated lives, finding their way to their very own happy ever after. For the last couple of years I'd been the main breadwinner, paying the bills while my husband, Ray, went back to college full time. To make ends meet, alongside writing novels, I'd also written for magazines and newspapers, for radio, short stories, travel guides, country house handbooks – in fact anything to make a living. Which was what led a friend, another writer, to send me a newspaper clipping about a publisher that was bringing out erotic fiction specifically written for women by women. My friend suggested that we both have a go at writing something. All they wanted was three chapters and a synopsis. What had we got to lose? After all, she reasoned, the sage advice given to all writers is to write about what you know. We were both married and we knew about sex. More than that, we knew about the sex we would enjoy given half a chance, which wasn't necessarily the same as the sex we were getting.

To be frank, writing erotica had never been up there on my 'Ten things to do before I die' list, but it was a new market, I needed to earn a living and I decided it was worth a shot – after all, what was the worst that could happen? They would reject my idea. What I hadn't bargained for was that it would help change my life for ever.

You'd think writing about sex would be easy, but when, after submitting my sample chapters, I was given a commission to write my first erotic novel and started work, I discovered it isn't.

You need to find ways to describe all the bits and pieces and goings on so that it doesn't sound like a public information film; and once you get past the labelling of parts you need to make it all sound sensual and romantic, and take your reader on a slow enjoyable journey towards a rip-snorting climax.

So no pressure then.

I kept a notebook alongside my keyboard with a whole collection of stick drawings in it, a visual aid to help me to work out what you could do given time, patience and no worries about a dodgy back – man woman, woman woman, man man, twosomes, threesomes, foursomes, orgy – as well as where all the bits go. While you can more or less guess what the business end is up to, where people put their arms, knees or elbows isn't always as clear, so you need to work it out, so that the mechanics are sorted and therefore more or less invisible, and your hero won't fall over while mid-fuck.

No one in erotica *ever* falls over unless they're being swept off their feet and ravaged. They don't get cramp, or the giggles, or trip over their pants while they're trying to take them off. No one passes wind and flaps the covers, laughing furiously. Zips never get stuck, everyone always

5

comes, and no one ever has a spotty bum. Humour and sex don't mix in erotic fiction, or so my new editor reliably informed me.

'Good erotic fiction should be like the best sex,' she said during one of our telephone conversations. 'A long, slow, satisfying build-up, hitting all the sweet spots, filling you with expectation, getting you more and more aroused, slowly bringing you closer and closer to the edge, making you gasp with pleasure, before finally taking you breathlessly to the grand finale. Erotic fiction should never let you down. Nobody in an erotic novel ever thought: let's get this over and done with, *X Factor*'s on at nine. Never, ever.'

The downside as a writer is that you need to have great sex in every chapter in lots of different, ever more exciting ways. In real life, not only is real sex not like that but also it doesn't need a plot. I'd been married a long time, and sex had long since slipped from something you were doing all the time to something squeezed into the to-do list, between cleaning out the guinea pig and collecting the kids from football practice. And unlike when you're writing about sex, during real sex you generally don't need to stop halfway through a really good bit to take the dog to the vet or nip out to buy the ingredients for your child's home economics bake-a-thon.

I hadn't got an office, so I was writing my first erotic novel on the family computer in a corner of the sitting room, squirrelling it away after each session in a desktop file labelled 'This year's tax receipts' and constantly reminding myself not to email it to my accountant. With a house full of teenagers the last thing I wanted was for them to read what I was writing, so I put an old-fashioned clothes horse around my desk, hung laundry all over it and told them it was to keep out the draught. My husband, although he knew what I was writing, never peeked. No one else in the family seemed to notice that the same towels and sheets hung there for weeks on end.

Halfway through the first book I stalled, stuttered and finally ran out of ideas. There were only so many ways our heroine could shed her clothes and gasp in breathless anticipation. Which was why Helen, Joan and I were all at Gabbie's, eating for England. They had volunteered to help me out.

'So it can be *anything*?' said Helen.

I nodded. 'Anything at all that you've ever fantasized about. Anything that you've always wanted to do, if you could do it without getting caught, and without risking disease or hurting anyone.'

'Or something we've already done,' said Gabbie, looking pointedly at Joan.

I nodded. 'I'm stuck,' I said. 'I really do need your help.'

'How tragic is that,' said Gabbie, laughing.

I was thinking they might come up with sex on a beach or in a sleeper train, or being ravished by a highwayman, but no: once they got going and were halfway through the Baileys, they were swapping real-life sexploits.

One had had sex on a cross-Channel ferry in the 1970s with a Frenchman she picked up in duty free, and when he told her that he wanted to see her again and asked for her name and telephone number, she lied through her eye teeth and told him her name was Freda and that she came from Margate.

Another had had a three-in-a-bed session with two builders who came to fix her parents' roof when she had been home from college in her twenties. Another admitted to a drunken lesbian romp while on a painting holiday in Tuscany – as she said, it wasn't something she particularly wanted to do again but she was glad she'd tried it. Which really did make it sound a bit like abseiling or hang-gliding – but she did add that it was incredibly refreshing to have sex with someone who actually knew where all your bits were.

I made notes – lots of notes.

'Oh, and then I went out with this guy, after I split up with Keith. Do you remember Stuart?' asked Gabbie. 'Big, sort of gingery?' She mimed tall with hair.

We all nodded.

'He used to like to spank me.'

I stared at her. 'And did you like it?'

Gabbie shrugged in a non-committal way. 'It was OK, I suppose. I think he was hoping it would turn me on, but it didn't. He kept saying that he'd really like to tie me up.'

'Oh, we tried that,' said Helen. 'The kids were at my mum's for the weekend. We did the whole thing: candlelit dinner, sexy underwear, silk scarf for a blindfold. Gav in this silk bathrobe I'd bought him for his birthday.' Helen grinned. 'God, I mean, he spent hours. It was fabulous. The only trouble was I wriggled so much that he couldn't get the bloody knots undone when we'd finished and had to cut me off the bed with a pair of scissors. I'd got a blindfold on, so it wasn't until he took it off I realized he'd used Molly's skipping rope. God, she was livid.'

'I blame *Cosmopolitan*,' said Gabbie, sucking chocolate out of her teeth.

'I've always fancied doing that,' I said, casually. 'Being tied up.'

'You should suggest it to Ray,' said Joan. 'Lots of men get off on that kind of thing. You know: helpless virgin, tied to a bed.' She rolled her eyes and waved her hands, squealing, 'Help, help,' in a very passable impression of Penelope Pitstop.

What I didn't tell them, and had never really admitted to myself until then, was that I'd fantasized about being tied up and spanked for years: not all the time, obviously, and it wasn't my only sexual fantasy, but it was there, carefully hidden and tucked at the back of my mind, and it was something I constantly revisited. The idea was a huge turn-on and had been for as long as I could remember – certainly long before my thoughts had turned to sex.

When it came to playing cowboys and Indians as a child, I had been the one who always volunteered to be held captive and tied to a tree. Want someone to hold hostage or whip until they give up the whereabouts of the cowboy encampment? Oooooo, oooo, yes please, that'd be me.

As I got older the fantasies became more explicit, and eventually sexual, and evolved to being put over someone's knee and soundly spanked, or being whipped with a riding crop, tied up or down, and made to do all sorts of interesting naughty things that my mother never told me about and certainly wouldn't approve of. But in all that time I had always kept these thoughts to myself. There was a part of me that was afraid to admit how much the idea excited me.

'Bob used to like me to tie him up,' said Joan conversationally, 'and thrash him with the cane on the feather duster. It wasn't really my kind of thing but he liked it. I used to find the feather duster upstairs in the bathroom and think: Oh, here we go again. He bought me a French maid's outfit the Christmas before we split ...'

In my fantasies the someone who did those wonderful things to me was always a broad-shouldered, dashingly handsome Prince Charming, who was good-looking in a clean-cut preppy kind of a way, and who was totally in control. He didn't say very much because, as is the way with fantasies, he always knew exactly what I wanted and when I wanted it, and was terribly good at giving it to me right on cue.

I'd be wearing high heels and I'd squeal in a girlie way, and after he had spanked me he would carry me over to a big four-poster bed and tie me down and blindfold me, before going to work with his knowing fingers and even more knowing tongue; then, when I was baying for more, he would make love to me, long and slow, until we both finally came. Visually it was a treat of rich colours, soft leather, huge four-poster beds, hairy chests and muscular torsos, and it was a fantasy that I kept on having, as I reworked the details.

I'd never told anyone about wanting to be spanked or whipped or tied down, because I was pretty much convinced that I was alone in thinking those kinds of things and finding a sexual charge in them. I assumed that they were definitely too weird to talk about, and certainly way too weird to do anything about. Yet here were my best friends talking about exactly that. Maybe what I wanted wasn't that unusual after all.

As I'd been taking notes, I was the only one who hadn't had a drink, and I drove home thinking through what the girls had told me. Looking in through the sitting-room window, I could see Ray slumped on the sofa watching TV in his tracksuit bottoms and a T-shirt. We'd been together for a long time; we had kids, dogs and a home together. Things weren't great between us. Money was tight, and while I was working every hour I could to try to keep our noses above water (he had been made redundant in a departmental rationalization and was now back at college, retraining), he refused to help by even thinking about a part-time job or helping round the house. As far as he was concerned, all that, and the children, were my responsibility, whether he was working or not. I was tired in lots of ways.

If you asked him, Ray would tell you with some pride that he was an old-fashioned man – a man who liked his wife at home. A proper family was what he called it. He'd probably have had a heart attack if I'd mentioned the whole tying-up thing. He was, and still is, a very practical man, a careful man; for him romance, luxury and adventurous sex were things other people had and I'd always felt he rather despised them.

As I unlocked the front door I thought about what Gabbie had said about sharing my fantasies with him, and realized with a growing certainty that it was probably too late.

Ray didn't even look away from the TV as I slipped off my coat. 'How did it go?' he asked.

'Oh, OK. I just want to get some of these notes down before I forget them,' I said.

He nodded, eyes still firmly fixed on the TV screen. With a sigh, I walked over to the computer, turned it on and got to work.

Over the next few weeks in every spare moment I worked on my first erotic novel. I reworked my friends' adventures and wove in all the things that turned me on. And more and more I had a sense of escaping into a fantasy world where anything was possible. I started to write all those things that had fuelled my fantasies for so long – and it was heady stuff. Most of them revolved around a tall, dark, handsome older man, who took control, and understood the heroine and what she needed and wanted, and gave them without question – with unconditional love and understanding. He was my Prince Charming, the alpha man of my fantasies.

I wondered, as I wrote, if that was what I thought I'd seen in Ray when I first met him. He was fifteen years older than me; I'd been working in a hotel for the summer when he asked me out. I'd seen him as capable, strong and silent. Things that at eighteen I had naively taken as positive qualities had, over the years, revealed themselves to be altogether less positive, and traits that probably a woman of his own age would have instantly recognized. He was stubborn and uncommunicative, and had, I suspected, chosen a much younger wife so that he could try to mould her into the woman he wanted. We got along fine until I wanted to grow up and have a life of my own.

Although I hadn't anticipated it, writing erotica was the perfect escape from the realities of a crumbling marriage. All those things that I'd never told anyone before, all those things I had longed to explore, finally had a place and a purpose.

I also spent a lot of time doing research on the internet, which up until that point I'd mostly used to buy shoes and books. Not altogether sure what I'd find, I was nervous, excited, sometimes shocked and sometimes delighted. The internet opened up a whole new world. I rapidly discovered that far from my being alone in my fantasies there was a whole sub-culture out there that I had known nothing about, and lots and lots of people who felt the same as I did. I wasn't so much relieved as stunned. And even better was that I found I had a name: I was a submissive.

In my fantasies, at least, I was a submissive – the one who gets spanked and tied up and gets all the attention. *Submissive*. I certainly didn't see myself as submissive in real life, but sexually I could see that it was a good fit.

Having sold my first attempt at writing female erotica, I wrote more – a lot more. The stuff that had fuelled my fantasies for years was suddenly fuelling my fiction and my finances; and having finally found a home for all those things I'd been dreaming about since my teens felt good. Having an outlet for my innermost thoughts helped paper over the cracks in my increasingly unhappy marriage, and I was having the best sex of my life, albeit on the page.

Over the next five years I wrote twelve novels and countless short stories. The books and short stories always involved some degree of bondage and submission, and other sexual shenanigans that can be loosely described as S&M (sadism and masochism) and BDSM (bondage, discipline, sadism and masochism), but in all that time, as I was writing about it and fantasizing about it, I never once tried any of it – not one single glorious black-leather, high-heeled, handcuffed moment of it. And Ray never read my books. Not one, ever.

Books, as Ray was eager to point out to anyone who would listen, were not his thing – and eventually, neither was I.

Finally the cracks just got too big and we separated. We were divorced within a year. It took me a while to get myself together, but after a few months I started, very tentatively, to date again. Fresh out of a long-term relationship, I wasn't altogether sure exactly how or where to begin. So after a few false starts I turned to the place where a lot of us begin again: internet dating websites.

I think we're often drawn to various incarnations of the devil we know – a type – and, having been married a long time, I certainly was. The men I dated after leaving Ray all seemed to have been cut from the same cloth. I was obviously doing something wrong. The men were all steady and practical, and I was still having married sex; I was just having it with new men.

Then along came Henry, my first attempt at trying to combine what passes for normal with some of the things I'd been fantasizing about.

After two glasses of house red and a light supper on our first weekend away together, I asked Henry if he'd ever thought about spanking anyone. You know – for fun. His eyes widened and his face took on an expression similar to the one I'd last seen on the face of a woman I'd offered a bacon butty, seconds before discovering she was a hard-line vegan.

Henry visibly stiffened and said, all outrage and horror, 'Good Lord, certainly not! What on earth do you think I am – some kind of a pervert?'

Well, yes, hopefully.

'Don't you have any fantasies?' I pressed, emboldened by strong drink and a nasty sinking feeling. The relationship had been pretty much doomed since lunchtime, when we'd been about to go Dutch on an uninspiring quiche and green salad when Henry had pointed out that actually I'd had a cappuccino and a sweet.

'Of course I have fantasies,' he said, 'but mostly they involve world peace and captaining the English cricket team during a one-day test at Headingley.'

Buddhists, what can I tell you?

So how did he feel about underwear? What sort of thing did he like? I asked, giving it one last shot and my voice dropping to a seductive purr.

'I haven't given it a lot of thought, to be perfectly honest.' He paused and then said, 'Something from Marks, probably.' I watched him slipping a bread roll into his pocket in case he got a bit peckish later. It wasn't the answer I'd hoped for, to be honest.

So that was it: I was a pervert. My first very tentative attempt at expressing what I wanted – fuelled by a little wine and a lot of nerve – had been thrown back in my face. It confirmed what I had feared: nice men didn't find this kind of stuff acceptable.

It was during that weekend that I decided it was time I found some way to let the genie out of the bottle and go in search of something else – something a little more rock and roll. I was in my mid-forties with a broken marriage and three children in their late teens and early twenties, and I wanted to try some of those things I had always dreamed of and been writing about, before it was too late. What had I got to lose?

It's a scary journey to start all on your own. What I needed was a guide: someone to help me find my way through a sexual landscape about which, despite several books, in reality I had absolutely no idea – and more to the point, someone who I felt I could trust enough to bring me out wiser but unscathed on the other side.

It had also occurred to me that maybe when I got to the point of experimenting I would chicken out, so I also needed someone with a sense of humour and a lot of patience: someone who wouldn't freak out if ultimately I put it all down to research.

I'm not sure I was setting out on a journey to look for a

happy-ever-after with anyone, but there definitely had to be a spark, that magic indefinable something between us. What I needed was a hero, a dominant man – referred to as a Dom in the BDSM world – who I could trust implicitly and who I liked, and who was prepared to help me, and spank me, and who I fancied. And we all know how very easy men like that are to find …

Then again, if I didn't try now, my fantasies would stay just that and I might as well settle down with someone like Henry and look forward to a lifetime of sensible pants and going Dutch.

When I arrived home after our weekend away I dumped him, put 'BDSM' into a search engine and watched the hits roll in. It is astonishing what you can find if you ask the right questions. There is everything you can ever want on the net and much more besides. Some of it in leather, some in plus sizes and an awful lot of it in America.

As I stared at the screen, flicking between websites, it occurred to me that I really needed to work out exactly what it was I was looking for. As research projects go I've had far worse. I made a list.

Chapter Two

'There is no more lively sensation than that of pain;
its impressions are certain and dependable, they
never deceive as may those of the pleasure women
perpetually feign and almost never experience.'
Marquis de Sade

A lot of reading, trawling and research later I took out a three-month membership on a well-known international BDSM website. I printed off a picture of Henry and taped it to the edge of my computer screen, just in case I weakened, and spent evenings browsing the site's personal ads for inspiration, trying to work up the courage to place an ad of my own. After all, that was why I'd joined, wasn't it? You couldn't contact anyone unless you had a profile on the site, so I couldn't email the men I thought looked interesting until I'd taken the plunge and posted something.

The trouble with real life, unlike fiction, is that you have no control over the outcome or how the plot develops. I was nervous of making the move, nervous of making a terrible mistake, scared that I'd be exposing myself to things that I had no understanding of with people I didn't know.

In the end, bizarrely, it was Henry who convinced me to get on with it. I'd read and re-read my profile, editing and adding to it until I'd almost lost sight of what I was trying to say, and was sitting with my finger hovering above the 'post' button for the fifth or sixth night in a row, trying to work up the courage to press it. I was about to have another go at editing my latest attempt when Henry rang and said he was sorry for whatever it was he'd done, and that he'd got tickets for an open-air concert at the weekend. Maybe I'd like to go with him?

And I almost said yes, except that he hadn't quite finished.

'I'd really like us to be friends, Sarah,' he said. 'The sex thing gets in the way a bit, don't you think? The tickets are thirty pounds each. I'm happy to take a cheque. I thought perhaps you could come over and pick me up.'

I didn't want a relationship with anyone who thought that sex got in the way. He was still talking when I pressed 'post'.

As I did, a little message popped up on the computer screen:

'Thank you for posting on our website. Your profile will appear on our system within twenty-four hours, although it is currently available for you to view and may still be edited. You may remove your profile or make it invisible at any time.'

My heart lurched. What the hell had I done?

'So what do you think?' said Henry.

'I think that I'm busy on Sunday,' I said, and hung up, still staring at the message on the screen.

Bloody hell! What if I attracted an axe-wielding psychopath? What if the website accidentally posted my real email address? Or my real name? Worse still, what if after all this whittling and worrying I didn't get a single reply?

A new message popped up alongside the first. 'Members with photos on their profiles attract more replies.'

I wasn't at all sure that I wanted to post a photo. What if someone recognized me? I flicked through the ones that had caught my eye – some had photos, but not all; some were full-faced, others pixellated, some were naked, some dressed. There didn't seem to be a norm: you posted what you were happy with.

I clicked through to my profile to read it one more time. I could always take it down.'Forty-something female novice submissive, with lots of imagination but no real-time experience, seeks a man to show her the ropes.'

There was a lot more but that was the gist of it. In the end I also posted a current photograph of myself on holiday in a sundress on a beach sipping a cocktail, with the face pixellated out.

Then I waited – and worried.

Maybe I'd made a mistake; maybe this was best kept as a fantasy. Maybe I'd just take my profile down before any harm was done. Maybe I'd give up on men and get some cats.

I was on tenterhooks all day, refusing to look at the site, wanting to peek at the website inbox but resisting the temptation.

That evening, when I'd finished my day's work, I opened up my account on the website. There were forty replies. I wasn't sure whether to be relieved or terrified.

Taking a deep breath to steady my nerves, I opened the first one: 'Hi, I saw your profile. Nice picture. My name is Craig and I'm a taxi driver and live just outside Cambridge. I'm into ...' It took about ten seconds for my anxiety to fade. These were real people, looking for the same thing as I was. There were some great emails among that first batch, including one from a woman, who emailed to offer advice.

The profiles were no longer nameless, faceless weirdos; they were people like me, and yes, they all had what other people might think of as unusual sexual tastes, but they were also looking for the same things as the rest of us – love, affection, sex, physical connections, understanding, companionship, someone to share things with, somewhere to belong.

I'd read dozens of other profiles before posting mine and I had composed an email to send to anyone who caught my eye. It didn't take me long to weed out the one-liners, the men who replied with a photo of their wedding tackle, and those who came across as illiterate, barking mad, wannabes or just plain weird. Though, oddly enough, in all the time when I met men from BDSM websites I met only one genuinely scary man – far fewer than on the straight sites I'd signed up to.

Over the next few days as the replies arrived I went through them all, reading every single one. I made a list of possible Doms to contact and ended up whittling those down to around a dozen before replying:

Thank you for replying to my recent ad.

I am a complete novice in this kind of lifestyle and I wondered whether it would be possible to make contact and/or talk?

I am deeply attracted to the idea of submission. I've written erotic fiction for several years and realized almost immediately that the thing that aroused me most was the idea of being submissive.

The trouble is I'm not sure how much of this is pure fantasy and how much I would, in real life, be able to cope with.

I am not a time-waster but I am naturally cautious while at the same time looking for a sane and safe and intelligent way to explore my sexuality. I wonder if you would be happy to talk to me?

Thank you for your time.

I look forward to hearing from you.

Over the next couple of months I spoke to almost all of the ones on my list and I met several. I was looking for someone whose kinks matched my own and who felt right. It was tricky – after all, mine were still all imaginary, untried kinks.

It's very odd meeting someone whose main shared interest isn't something like gardening or films but what you like sexually. Before my first meeting I was a bag of nerves and sat in the car wondering if I should just text him and say I'd chickened out.

We had arranged to meet for coffee. Heading for the café, I half expected somebody in black leather and studs.

Instead, I met a lovely man who was very keen to spank me and lock me in a large dog cage overnight. He was quietly spoken with charming manners, taught at a university and advised me not to rush and to enjoy the journey. While it was obvious from the second we met there was not a molecule of chemistry between us, he offered me a trial run, and to be a listening ear if I ever felt the need.

Later I met a pilot who liked to write obscenities on his partner in felt tip and then flog them; a fireman, who I really thought might be it, until he spent the whole time we were having coffee talking about anal sex; and a librarian, who was an absolute sweetie and with whom I've remained friends, and who was into pony girls and showed me pictures of his ex-wife dressed up in a harness, saddle, bells and buckles – she looked fabulous, although to be fair she was more Shetland pony than Arab filly. But none of them felt right, and I needed it to feel right for me to even consider taking the next step.

'How do you feel about handcuffs?' asked my lunch date as he reached across the table to top up my glass.

'In what way?' I asked, trying hard to sound nonchalant. The pub I'd chosen to meet at was busy; there were other people within earshot. This was the third Dom I'd met in the last couple of weeks.

'Well,' he said, moving his chair in closer and leaning towards me across the table. 'I've got quite a collection of restraints – everything from vintage shackles right through to some lovely little stainless-steel cuffs that I bought in the Far East while I was on holiday there last year. They've got little tiny rows of teeth on the inside.' He mimed. 'I'm not a great fan of cable ties. Actually, I've brought a few of my favourites along with me in the back of the car,' he continued enthusiastically. 'Maybe you'd like to take a little look after we've eaten?'

I turned my attention back to my salad, decided not to bother with the wine, and instead counted down the minutes till my mobile pinged to announce an incoming text message. I'd arranged for Joan to text me. If it was going well I'd text back a pre-agreed reply. Anything else, including silence – particularly silence, and she would call out the cavalry. If I felt the need to escape, it was an easy get-out-of-jail-free card.

I'd read the incoming text, look concerned, and say something along the lines of 'Oh no! Look, I'm so sorry, but I've really got to go. I'll ring you this evening/some time later/the very second Hell freezes over.' And I could be up and away without either of us losing face.

Right on cue the phone pinged. I whipped it out of my handbag and rearranged my face into an expression of deep regret.

'Don't tell me, you have to go,' said the man with a sigh before I had a chance to say anything. 'What is it? What is it that I'm doing wrong?'

Where to begin? Showing me pictures of handcuffs you've known and loved while we waited to be shown to a table? Being a foot shorter and twenty years older than you said on your profile? Asking the waitress for the cheapest thing on the menu and then adding, 'You didn't want a starter, did you?' Turning up in a particularly nasty beige Bri-Nylon car coat?

If I hadn't been so damned polite, I would have pretended I had no idea who you were and just carried on walking.

I smiled and rested my hand very lightly on his. 'A lot of this is about chemistry, isn't it? And let's be honest, there isn't any, and I think you know straight away, don't you?' I said, in a voice that implied he was the kind of person who was sensitive to that kind of thing. 'You're a lovely man, but not my sort of man. I'm sure you'll find someone who really appreciates you for who you are.'

He sighed again. 'You're right, and besides, if I'm perfectly honest, love, when I first saw you walk in I thought you were a bit long in the tooth for me; and with a bit too much meat on you, if you get my drift. I like my women quite a bit younger really. And slimmer.'

And probably sold with a foot pump, I thought with a fixed smile, as I got up, waved *au revoir* to Manacle Man, left my half of the bill on the table and headed home, mentally crossing another possibility off my would-be-Dom list.

I was beginning to feel that I was looking for something that didn't exist. But then, just when I was thinking of giving up, I got an email from Max.

Chapter Three

'The imagination is the spur of delights ...
all depends upon it, it is the
mainspring of everything.'
Marquis de Sade

Max had been one of the Doms on my original list of twelve from the very first batch of contacts. In fact, I had contacted him directly after reading his profile and posting mine, but he had been out of the country on business on a four-month contract and, after expressing his regret, said that much as he'd like to help, long-distance Domming really wasn't his bag. He promised to be in touch as soon as he arrived home, assuming that I hadn't found someone in the meantime, and he was very happy to talk and answer any questions I had, whether I had found someone or not. He wished me luck.

Max was a few years older than me, around six feet tall, with dark hair shot through with grey. On his profile he came across as witty, confident and warm. It was well written, readable, and in that happy land between a one-liner and being way too long. He also sounded sane, reasonable and, broadly speaking, as if he was looking for the same kind of things as I was. To be honest, he had slipped my mind, so I was really pleased when, after Manacle Man, his email arrived.

Dear Sarah

Thank you for your email. Apologies for the delay in getting back to you, but I didn't arrive back in the UK until late last week.

First of all let me say I'm honoured that you contacted me.

In answer to the first part of your email, yes of course it is possible to talk. May I suggest that you use the private email address [provided] or if you prefer you can ring me on my mobile [which he included]. This is a mobile number for obvious security reasons, but should we decide to extend our contact then I'd be more than happy to give you my landline number.

As I am sure you realize, there are a vast range of possibilities existing in the Dom/sub world and it's important that you try and find someone with wants and needs that are similar to your own. It's better to wait for the right fit than be unhappy or uncomfortable with your choices.

You have obviously gathered that I am a Dom.

My view on the Dom/sub relationship is hard to sum up in a few paragraphs, but basically I don't believe that subs should be subjected to continual physical pain or abuse. I'd be lying if I said these don't have a part, but there is much more to be gained in other areas, particularly in the mind.The fact that you write erotic fiction suggests that you already understand the power of the imagination – and I suspect that the anticipation of future events could be important to you. I would obviously be interested in reading some of your work.

There are many ways that fantasy can become reality, but as you have suggested, finding a sane and safe way to express and explore it is often hard. Many people would expect to move forward quickly; however, I suggest that we move at your pace. I do have some fundamental rules of engagement – but let's talk first and then we can discuss what, if anything, comes next.

Kind regards

Max

He sounded nice, interesting, articulate. Just reading the email gave me a funny little buzz of anticipation, although I had to remind myself that this wasn't a fantasy, and nor was Max a character in one of my books; this was potentially the real thing, with a real man. I emailed Max back with a list of questions. He replied, taking everything point by point, and then suggested that it might be much easier if we talked on the phone.

Easier yes. Easier actually to dial the number? No.

I sat at my desk and stared at his number for a while, wondering whether I dared ring or not. The thing was he sounded so right that I'd be a fool not to ring; but if he wasn't, given how many people I'd met and how disappointed I'd been, how was I going to feel? What if he spoke with a high-pitched nasal twang? What if he was like Manacle Man? What if he was not at all as I imagined him? In lots of ways Max felt like the last roll of the dice before I crept back to normal land with my tail between my legs.

I dialled his number but couldn't quite bring myself to press 'call'. Lots of what ifs flitted through my mind, but the bottom line was I'd never know what he was like until we spoke. Finally I pressed the button.

The phone rang at the other end – once, twice, three times, four. How long before hanging on for the pick-up came across as desperate? Maybe he wasn't in; maybe I'd dialled the wrong number.

'Hello,' said a deep, cultured male voice.

'Hello, Max?' I said. 'It's Sarah.'

'Sarah, great to hear from you. I'm really pleased you called,' he said. 'I was just thinking about you.'

Any nervousness I had had about talking to him evaporated within seconds. Max's voice was warm and tinged with good humour. He was easy to talk to from the first sentence, answered everything I asked him without hesitation, and made me laugh. It also soon became clear during our first phone call that he was many, many other things besides a Dom.

He liked to cook, liked the theatre, films, travel, books and music, but that natural need to be in charge and take control had informed his whole life and the choices he had made. He ran a successful business, he was confident and articulate, and while his sexual preferences weren't something he broadcast in his everyday life they were something he was completely at ease with. He was a breath of fresh air.

Over the next couple of weeks we spoke most evenings, until it became obvious that the next step was meeting or calling it a day.

'So,' said Max at the end of a marathon session on the phone, 'would you like to meet?'

'Yes, I'd like that.'

'But?' he prompted. I knew he'd heard it in my voice.

We'd got on really well on the phone and chatted for hours, but I was worried that when we met we might not be what the other had imagined. I told him so.

'There's only one way to find out. But before we meet, we need to talk about how things progress from here. I want you to understand that, for me, BDSM is a real-life thing –'

'I know,' I began. 'We've talked –'

'You need to understand what you're getting into.' Max sounded cool and businesslike. 'There are rules of engagement that we both need to observe when we play together. I've drawn up a contract.'

'Are you serious?' I said. I'd seen and written contracts in BDSM novels but I wasn't sure that they existed in real-life BDSM relationships.

'Contracts are a big part of the BDSM life. It's for my protection as much as yours. Have you thought about how one of your friends would react if she came in and found you tied up and me horsewhipping you?'

I hadn't.

'The contract shows that you've given me consent. I know we've talked about the things that turn us both on, but we also need to discuss the point beyond which you are not prepared to go, and the things you find unacceptable.'

'Surely those things are obvious?'

He laughed. 'You would have thought so, wouldn't you, but it's better if they're spelled out and down on paper.'

I said it all sounded a bit formal.

'It is,' Max said. 'We're moving this up a gear. You need to learn to be frank and honest with me – the relationship between Dom and sub is far more open and intimate than one between straight couples. And you'll need to choose safe words.'

I'd written about safe words in my books, so I knew what they were: they're used between BDSM partners to stop any activity that is going too far. Max wanted me to choose three: one that would tell him that everything was OK, should he ask, one for 'slow down' and one for 'stop'.

For the first time since we'd started to talk on the phone I felt uneasy and nervous, and he picked that up. 'It's OK,' he said. 'I know you're unsure about what you can cope with, but we can only find your limits by trial and error. We'll take it really slowly. And for my part of the bargain I promise I'll keep you safe, answer your questions as best I can and try to give you all the things you're looking for.'

'And all this is in writing?'

'It is,' he said. 'Also when we're playing I will expect you to give me total and complete obedience.'

I took a deep breath. 'Really?'

'It's not negotiable,' he said.

'Bloody hell! I need to think about that.'

Max laughed. 'OK. Well, I'm not going anywhere. You OK?'

'I'm fine. I suppose I'm just coming to realize what a big thing this can be.'

'It changes your life for ever,' he said. 'I'll talk to you tomorrow.'

After I had hung up I read and re-read everything he had sent me.

Max had been married in his early twenties and had adult children, and was separated from his long-term girl-friend, Abby, with whom he had had a daughter. She was called Ellie and she was six. He and Abby had parted amicably and he was still in contact with her, and despite Abby moving halfway across the country he saw Ellie regularly. He also had a good relationship with his ex-wife and his grown-up children. He seemed ideal, but endless phone conversations and half-a-dozen emails were certainly no guarantee that he was what I was looking for, nor that he was telling the truth: anyone can be anyone on the phone.

What did I do next? I went downstairs, made a mug of tea and then picked the phone up and dialled his number. Max picked up on the second ring.

'Hello,' he said. 'That was quick.'

'Can we meet?' I said. 'Before I bottle out.'

'Of course,' Max said. 'How about lunch next week?'

Max insisted I choose the place and the time, so that I would feel safe. The rules were that I picked somewhere very public but with the potential for privacy – some-where where, if we saw each other and didn't like what we saw, we could smile and walk on. No games here with text messages. Max said if we didn't click he would have no problem with either of us calling it a day and that I shouldn't either. And lastly I should choose somewhere where we could actually get a decent lunch if we liked the look of each other, although he was quick to remind me that at this point there were no strings.

I suggested we meet outside Norwich Cathedral, which wasn't that far from where I lived. I'd worked in Norwich for four years at the end of the 1990s and still had lots of friends there; the shopping is fabulous, and there are some great places to eat in and loads of places to wander round – all of which meant I had places to go to and people to see if the meeting with Max didn't work out.

So it seemed a good choice. We could take a look around inside the cathedral and talk in relative privacy. There were a couple of good restaurants and some nice cafés all within easy walking distance. Being a staunch atheist, Max thought the cathedral was a great idea.

At this point I was feeling good, a bit nervous maybe, a little bit excited, but in a good way, and certainly in control. Then Max sent me another email and the balance of power began to subtly shift:

Dear Sarah

It was good to speak this evening and I'm delighted that we are finally going to meet. In future if we continue with our liaison you will call me Sir unless given permission to do otherwise. In the hearing of other people you may call me Max.

When we meet you will wear a white blouse, loose-fitting dark skirt and high-heeled shoes.

You will also wear clean white underwear and black stockings. You may choose whether to wear a suspender belt or not; if you make the wrong choice you will be punished.

You may wear a suitable coat.

You will measure the size of your neck and wrists and let me know the measurements so that I can have a collar and cuffs made for you.

You may be physically examined to see if you complied exactly with my instructions.

Oh yes, I nearly forgot: I'm really looking forward to meeting you at last. See you next week.

With kind regards

Max

As I read and I re-read his email, I was torn between thinking just who the hell does he think he is and being really excited. Finally, this was my chance to try this stuff for real, while another part of me – some people would probably say the saner, more sensible part of me – was extremely nervous. Was this really what I wanted? Physically examined? *Was he mad?*

There was still time to back out. Meeting him didn't imply any kind of commitment, I reminded myself. I'd met enough men on straight dating sites and walked away without a second thought to know that it was no big thing, and in essence at least this was no different, but that wasn't how it felt at all.

I barely slept. The next morning I re-read the email and emailed back. What I didn't do was comment on any of Max's conditions or agree to them. I needed to take this one step at a time.

… I'm excited about the whole idea; the combination of imagining and apprehension and excitement is a heady one. I am also very nervous about meeting up and moving this from a fantasy towards a reality, but would very much like to try. You do know that I'm just as likely to run a mile, don't you?

His reply excited me even more:

One of the joys of being a submissive is the anticipation of things to come, the emotion produced by fear of the unknown. I will always try and describe what will happen to you before doing it. This way you will experience double the pleasure, first in your imagination and then in reality. See you soon.

Max

So this was it. Finally. I switched off my computer and went back downstairs. It felt as though I was teetering on the brink of something huge.

Chapter Four

'There is no fulfilment that is not made
sweeter for the prolonging of desire.'
Jacqueline Carey, Kushiel's Dart

I was early. For some reason the outer doors into the cathedral porch were locked when I got there. It was pouring with rain, and my feet – crammed into high heels that I'd only ever worn once, for two hours, to a friend's wedding – were wet and cold and hurt like hell. On the walk up from the car park a freak gust of wind had turned my umbrella inside out and wrecked it, and I wasn't altogether sure exactly how waterproof my coat was. This was not at all how I'd imagined my first meeting with Max. I was nervous enough without going from coiffured to quagmire in the space of a short walk.

Having wandered up and down the street a few times, I finally managed to find some shelter from the rain, but not from the biting wind, although at least I had a view of the main doors.

My feet ached and I could feel my carefully constructed appearance rapidly dissolving – hair, make-up, composure: going, going, gone. A party of Asian tourists trekked past me with their guide. Wide eyed and curious, wrapped up in colourful cagoules and peculiar hats, they nodded and smiled in my direction, holding up umbrellas over their cameras to take pictures of me sheltering, wet and dripping, under one of the stone arches. Maybe they thought I was performance art.

The minutes ticked by. I was getting more anxious with every passing second. I glanced down at my watch. Max and I had agreed to meet at 11.00 a.m. As I said, I'd arrived early – I'm always early. It was almost ten past. I found myself peering into the faces of strangers under umbrellas as they scuttled by. I have a problem with people who are late.

Maybe Max wasn't going to show up after all, maybe he had just been stringing me along, maybe he was just a fantasist: my brain cheerily offered all kinds of explanations for his tardiness, each darker than the previous one. With a growing sense of disappointment, I considered my options. Up until that point I hadn't realized exactly how high my expectations had been.

If it had been sunny I probably wouldn't have minded waiting around a little longer, but I'd had enough. Another two minutes and if he hadn't shown up I'd head off for lunch on my own, a little older, wiser and considerably wetter. Maybe my hopes were too high, but I was deeply disappointed that Max had stood me up. During our email exchanges and telephone conversations he had seemed genuine and genuinely interested. I was just turning to leave when someone touched me on the shoulder.

'Off somewhere? You look like you could use a coffee,' said a familiar voice.

I glanced round and looked into a pair of amused blue eyes 'Max?'

He grinned from under the shelter of a large black umbrella. He was slightly out of breath. 'I'm so sorry I'm late. I got caught up in an accident on the ring road,' he said. 'Did you get my text?'

I shook my head. Why in heaven's name hadn't it occurred to me to check my phone? How stupid was that?

'Are you OK?'

I nodded.

'Good.' Still smiling, he reached out and brushed a stray, very damp strand of hair off my face. 'Come on. There's a café just round the corner. Let's go and get warmed up.' With that he took my arm and we made our way out of the cathedral precincts and across the road. 'You look like you need towelling off. We could find a shop –'

I shook my head. 'No, it's OK. I'll be fine, really.'

'You're sure?'

It felt easy and very natural. I felt comfortable with Max from the moment we met and there was definitely a crackle of mutual attraction – the chemistry thing, that thing I'd been looking for unsuccessfully on straight dates. I smiled.

He grinned at me. 'Good to meet you at long last,' he said.

We hurried across the road, huddling together under his umbrella. Max opened the café door for me, found a table and, when the waitress arrived, ordered for both of us, which I found a bit unsettling.

'Is that a Dom thing? What if I don't like what you've ordered?' I said in an undertone as the girl left.

'But you do,' he said.

'You can't know that.'

'Trust me.'

'I could be gluten intolerant.'

'And are you?' he asked, his expression amused.

'No.'

'Well, in that case you'll be able to enjoy your cake, won't you?'

I didn't say anything; I just raised my eyebrows. After a second or two Max held up his hands in surrender. 'OK. It was easy. When you came in, the first thing you did was look in the cake cabinet, and I noticed the cakes your eyes lingered on.'

I laughed. 'Lingered on?'

His smile widened. 'Well, OK – lusted after. It's OK, I really like a woman with a healthy appetite. And every time we've spoken on the phone, at some point during the conversation you've mentioned needing a cup of tea.'

Was I that obvious? And was it that simple? I really hoped not. I didn't want the Dom/sub relationship to be some trick or sleight of hand.

A few minutes later the waitress reappeared with our order: a pot of Earl Grey for him and good old builders' tea for me. Alongside it on the tray was a slice of lemon drizzle cake.

Max raised his eyebrows in a silent question. He was right. He'd ordered my favourite cake, although I wasn't about to tell him that. He laughed as he poured tea for us both.

'Come on, eat up and stop bristling,' he said. 'Would you prefer to stay here and talk or shall we go for a walk? It looks like the rain is easing up and there's a really nice little restaurant which a friend recommended in the lanes.'

'In these shoes?' I said ruefully. 'Isn't there any chance I can be kinky in flats?'

He threw back his head and laughed. 'I'm sure I saw a shoe shop round the corner. We'll go there first, if you like. I prefer any pain I inflict to be deliberate rather than accidental.'

I looked at him and smiled. 'It's fine. I've got spare shoes in my bag,' I said.

'OK, in that case we'll walk, then, shall we?'

I nodded.

Max was very upright, with broad shoulders, and his demeanour was slightly stiffer than I'd expected from talking to him on the phone, although there was no mistaking the mischief in his eyes. There was a slightly leonine quality about him – he wore his hair swept back off his face, he was heavily set, with a web of laughter lines picking out large blue eyes. While we were in the café I noticed his hands, which were large and very still, something I noticed particularly because I gesticulate all the time and find it almost impossible to talk without moving my hands. He wasn't handsome in any traditional sense but his features were strong, even and nicely made, and it was obvious from the way he moved that he looked after himself and worked out.

We settled into easy conversation. We talked about our journeys, my job, his trip to Europe, the weather, my choice of footwear, the tourists, the cake – all very comfortable and conversational, but it was impossible to ignore the undercurrent of expectation that was beginning to build up between us.

'So,' he said, 'have you done as I asked?'

I stared at him; the words made my heart flutter. I nodded.

'Is that a yes?' he pressed.

'Yes,' I said, not quite meeting his eyes; God, this felt so tricky. I was aware that this was the moment of transition when potentially it all finally began to become real.

'Good. You understand that if we continue with this arrangement you will call me Sir, but not today. Today you can call me Max, but if we take this further it is one of the few things that are non-negotiable. Do you understand?'

I nodded.

'And I want you to answer me with a word, not a gesture, from now on. So, are you wearing stockings and suspenders or did you decide on hold-ups?' he asked.

I was wearing stockings and suspenders, not wanting to risk the possibility that the hold-ups wouldn't.

Max raised his eyebrows. 'Well?' he said.

'Stockings and suspenders,' I said, glancing around to see who might have overheard our conversation, feeling my colour rise. 'I'm finding this hard. I've never done anything like this before.'

'I know,' he said, and then he took an envelope from his jacket pocket and slid it across the table towards me. 'Do you remember what I said?'

How could I possibly forget? I'd read and re-read the email so many times that I could practically recite it in my sleep. I stared down at the envelope, deciding to play dumb.

'Let me refresh your memory, Sarah. If you make the wrong choice, then you will be punished.'

'And if I make the right choice?'

'If you make the right choice, then you will be rewarded.' His expression was neutral but I could see the amusement in his eyes. 'Why don't you open it while I try and attract our waitress's attention?'

I picked the envelope up, peeled it open and took out the card inside. Glancing down, I read the words neatly written in block capitals across the centre. I could feel Max watching me.

According to the card I should have been wearing hold-ups and my punishment for not doing so was to be spanked. Soon. At a time and place of my choosing.

I looked across into Max's face and from him up into the face of the waitress, who was standing by the table holding a pen and pad.

Max was smiling, triumphant. 'More tea?' he asked.

Chapter Five

'Sex is as important as eating or drinking and we
ought to allow the one appetite to be satisfied with
as little restraint or false modesty as the other.'
Marquis de Sade

Max and I spent the afternoon together. We ate lunch. We
walked round the castle. We explored the shops. We talked
and talked and talked, and at no time did Max mention
the card or my punishment. As he walked me back to my
car he shook my hand and kissed me on the cheek.

'Call me when and if you're ready,' he said as a final
farewell.

As I watched him walking away, I wondered exactly
what I'd started. Was I ready? It felt as if this was one of
those now-or-never moments. Taking a deep breath, I took
the phone out of my bag and scrolled down to his number.
He was still so close that I could hear the phone when it
started ringing. I saw him pull the phone out of his pocket,
saw him look at the caller display, saw him smile as he
turned back to look at me.

'Hello,' he said. 'Fancy it being you.'

* * *

A week later and Max was wearing much the same expression as he pulled a mask down over my eyes. The mask was nothing threatening, a black, silky little number, not dissimilar to the kind of thing they hand out free on airlines.

'Are you OK?' he asked, as the lights went out.

I nodded.

'I'm afraid that's not good enough, Sarah. From now on you have to say "Yes, Sir." Or come to that, "No, Sir."'

Have to? I pulled a face – preposterous. But this was supposed to be me being punished, and earlier we had signed a contract, designed to protect us both, and yes, I had signed up to calling him Sir.

'I'm waiting,' he said. His tone was unmistakably crisper.

'Yes, Sir,' I mumbled. It felt ridiculous and made me feel stupidly self-conscious. Today was the day when I was supposed to be receiving my punishment for not wearing hold-ups, and in a perverse way, my reward – for being bad by some contrived set of fantasy rules that we had set in motion.

'Very good,' Max said. 'It will get easier, I promise you, until in the end it'll be second nature.'

I very much doubted that. I stood still – possibly the stillest I've ever been in adulthood – blindfolded, wondering what would come next.

'So here we are at last,' murmured Max.

He wasn't alone in feeling that way and I wondered if he had any idea just how much I had agonized – once the giddiness of our first face-to-face meeting had evaporated

– about whether to meet him again or just ring and call the whole thing off. I also wasn't altogether sure how I felt about being punished for a made-up crime. I was heading into completely uncharted water here.

Since we had met for lunch Max and I had spoken every night on the phone.

I had no questions left – only a decision. He had sent me a contract the evening after our first meeting so that I might have a better idea of what to expect if I took it to the next stage. He had also mailed me a long list of book and film titles and links to websites, so that I could find out more about the reality of the lifestyle. But, as he said, he couldn't make that final decision for me; nor would he attempt to coerce or force me into making it. I was always free to change my mind. If I was unsure about taking the next step it was better to walk away and take more time to think about it than to commit to something I was uncomfortable with – and it would be a commitment.

He was keen to impress on me that for him BDSM was not a joke. If I didn't want to abide by the rules that was fine, but then he wasn't the Dom for me. He also pointed out that once I had taken the step there was no going back. You couldn't unknow something – and it had the potential to change my life and the way I looked at relationships for ever.

So not exactly a lightweight thing, then, I'd joked. This wasn't quite what I'd imagined when I'd fantasized about being tied up and spanked.

For once Max didn't laugh. 'No, that's true. It changes you,' he said. 'You need to bear that in mind before you go any further. And yes, it's a game and in some ways it's just role play, but getting involved in BDSM is not without consequences, and the effects and the pay-off are real.'

The contract itself had come as no great surprise. Contracts are common currency and typical for people involved in a BDSM relationship in fiction. I'd written them myself for several books, and the ones I had drawn up for my novels had been a good deal more extreme and a lot pervier. The difference, of course, was that this one wasn't a work of fiction for some long-limbed, doe-eyed virgin. It was about me.

CONTRACT

On this _th day of _____, 20 ___, I, _____, hereafter referred to as the submissive, offer myself to Max _____, hereafter known as her Master, for His pleasure in a BDSM relationship defined in detail as follows.

The submissive understands that her Master is a strict Dominant, and that she is a willing submissive masochist to be used for His pleasure. The submissive expects and longs for the Domination of her Master and is willing to endure any punishments deemed appropriate by her Master. The submissive hereby grants permission to her Master to inflict any punishment that He may deem appropriate to the submissive totally for His enjoyment and the pleasure.

The submissive will refer to her Master as 'Sir' at all times when they are together, unless instructed to do otherwise.

The submissive will not speak until spoken to or given express permission to speak and will be respectful in her conversation and comments.

The submissive will be under her Master's complete and total control and will immediately obey and comply with any order or instruction given to her with the full joy of knowing she is His property and His to use however He chooses.

If the submissive displeases or disobeys her Master in any way she expects to be punished in any way He so chooses, as necessary for her inappropriate actions.

The submissive also agrees not to make any change in her physical appearance without the prior approval of her Master.

The submissive agrees to full participation in any and all activities her Master desires as she does not know the extent of her limits with Him at this point and desires to learn how complete is her submission. These activities may include but not be confined to:

Bondage of short or long duration

Pain threshold

Nipple and other clamps

The use of toys

The use of any safe stimulation chosen by her Master

Any and all sexual activities that her Master may wish to partake in, which involve the total use of the submissive for His physical pleasure

In return for her complete compliance and obedience the submissive expects the following:

The right to use safe words or signals if she finds the play to go past her as yet unknown limits

That her Master and the submissive will have open and honest communication with each other so that she may learn her limits

The knowledge that her Master may reward her for good behaviour and compliance

Her Master will practise safe sex

Her Master will be responsible for the submissive's safety during all play and ensure that no permanent harm or damage will befall her

Name:
  Signed:
  Safe words:

We had talked about a sex clause. Despite fancying Max and feeling an unmistakable chemistry between us, I wanted to wait a little while until we knew each other better before having full sex – which with hindsight seems crazy – but I thought it was telling, and certainly made me trust him more, that he'd put a line through it without comment.

We could reconsider it at a later date, he said.

I nodded, although I didn't think either of us believed we would wait for long.

'You know that this contract is complete nonsense, don't you?'

'Not if you believe in it,' Max said calmly, picking up the pen and handing it to me.

I took another look. 'Can't we do what we're going to do without this?'

'No,' said Max. 'There are some things that you can pick and choose, Sarah, but this isn't one of them. If you don't sign it we don't take the next step.'

'But no one is going to enforce this.'

'They don't have to. It's for our benefit. If you don't trust me enough to sign it, Sarah, that's fine, but we don't play without it.'

I read it again. 'You're serious?'

'Never more so.'

I was torn between frustration, amusement, annoyance and apprehension. If I signed it, it was a sign that I took all this seriously and that we were moving forward. Surely after I'd come this far it was what I wanted.

'It's mad,' I said.

'Possibly.'

I agonized. When it came right down to it, I realized I was also afraid. Afraid of him? Of me? It was hard to be specific.

'You have to trust me. I'll look after you and I promise not to do anything to you that you can't cope with. I promise ...'

And he was right: if we wanted to move this on, then I had to trust him. Looking back, I have no idea why I believed him, but I did.

The contract was currently sitting on my office desk, all signed and sealed. Even as I'd added my signature there was still a part of me that thought it didn't really count and that, when you got right down to it, it was all completely crazy. I knew full well that in reality no one could hold me to a contract like this if I didn't want to comply with the conditions.

As I passed the pen over to Max, as if reading my mind, he looked across at me and said, 'Sarah, this contract is only as meaningful as you make it. I want you to understand that for me this isn't some kind of joke. Have you read the list of hard limits that I sent you?'

I had. Hard limits are areas of engagement between a Dominant and a submissive which are off-limits: no-go areas. Both subs and Doms can have them, list them, discuss them and expect their limits to be respected. Once again they were things I had read about before, but they had never related to me, or anyone or anything I'd actually been involved in. It was the last part of the bargain to be sealed before we could play:

No breath or underwater play
No animals, no children or minors
No electrical play
No scat
No suspension
No needles, blood or blades

Max asked me if there was anything I wanted to add before we both signed. I said I wanted to include no photographs and no video, and also reserve the right to add things to the list as I discovered more about the lifestyle. Max agreed, happy to accept that our contract was a work in progress, and watched while I added the clause.

Standing there now, blindfolded and alone, it occurred to me that that still left an awful lot of things that weren't hard limits. An awful lot of things that Max could do to me and not break our contract.

'I'm scared,' I murmured.

'I will keep you safe,' Max said. 'I promise.'

I swallowed hard, trying to quell my nerves. I was trembling.

The room was still and there was complete silence. Seconds ticked by. I was tempted to ask Max what was going to happen next. What he was playing at? What was he going to do to me? Hadn't he said that he would tell me what he was going to do? Despite being desperate to say something, I was also painfully aware that less than half an hour earlier I'd signed up to the 'not speaking unless spoken to while we were together' thing and I'd already broken the rule once. This was going to be so much trickier than I had imagined. At forty plus I'd never willingly kept quiet about anything in years. I had an opinion and a wisecrack for every occasion.

It was so quiet now that I swear I could hear my heart beating. Where the hell was Max? My senses struggled to reach out from beyond the mask, struggling to track him down. Had he slipped away? Gone home? Had I blown it already with the whole Sir thing?

Finally, after what seemed like an age, I heard Max moving and sensed him circling around until he was standing behind me, so close that I could feel his breath on my neck. I shivered.

We were standing in my sitting room, and – if I had taken my mask off – I would have been able to see us both reflected in the mirror that hung above the fireplace. Being unable to see meant that I was totally focused on every sound and every sensation. That alone was heady stuff. Max stroked my cheek and I sighed with a mixture of relief and an intense abstract rush of desire.

'There, not so bad, is it?' Max said. I didn't know what to say. It was much, much worse and much, much better than I'd imagined. My whole body felt as if it was awake and waiting, tingling, every molecule listening for whatever it was that was coming next. Excitement, expectation – it was hard to pin down exactly what it was that I was feeling.

Max's fingers moved down across my shoulder to the zip of my dress. Very slowly he began to undo it. I felt my pulse quicken and swallowed hard to quell the heady mix of nerves and exhilaration. He pressed his lips into the curve of my neck, to my spine, sending wave after wave of tingling sensations through me.

He ran his fingers through my hair, tugging at it, toying with it, moving my head around. I wasn't sure if he expected me to resist or go with it. I started to tremble, adrenaline coursing through my veins like champagne as his lips brushed my naked shoulders, breathing me in. I felt the zip working its way lower; Max was unhurried, his fingers deft and confident.

I realized I was holding my breath. We hadn't kissed since we'd met, at least not in a sexual way – our lunch at the restaurant had ended with a handshake and the kind of peck on the cheek I'd give to a maiden aunt. Those kisses on my shoulders felt as if they were seared into my skin.

Doms didn't kiss their subs on the mouth, he'd said. It had made sense then, but now? I was going to say it felt weird to be undressed by a man I hadn't kissed but actually when you got right down to it the whole damned thing was weird.

'Don't try and rationalize it,' Max had said, when I'd been trying to work out, and justify, why I wanted to do this. 'You'll drive yourself crazy. Just accept that this is what you like, and want, and that it is a part of your nature. This is what you need, Sarah. It's not strange or weird; it's just part of human sexuality. I can give you what you want.'

Easy for him to say. Although I was beginning to realize that he was right. I hadn't felt so alive in years. I felt like a present being slowly and skilfully unwrapped by him. This was what I had written about for so many years; this was what I had dreamt about. Finally here I was. This was for real.

As Max's fingers brushed my skin, I could almost see the sensations in my head, like pinpricks of light exploding in a sea of velvety darkness.

I shivered as the zipper slipped down another inch or two more, stunned by how long he was taking. How long was it since someone had taken the time to do this properly? My emotions seesawed back and forth. I wondered if Max was expecting me to call a halt. The safe words we had agreed on were: gold for 'everything is OK'; silver for 'please slow down'; lead for 'stop, stop *now*'.

He was taking it oh-so-slowly, the slightest touch of his fingers, lips and tongue making me gasp.

Gold, silver, lead: I repeated the words over and over in my head. It would be so easy to stop this before it even began, but I didn't want to stop – far from it. I wanted it so much. I had waited so long to play this game for real. Behind the mask, crazily, I closed my eyes and tried to remember the last time I had felt this excited, this turned on or this bloody nervous.

Max eased the dress off my shoulders and let it slip down over my arms before letting it slither to the floor. Despite the mask I reddened, extraordinarily self-aware, imagining his expression as he looked me up and down, imagining what he could see.

He made a soft throaty noise of approval. 'Nice,' he purred. 'Very nice.'

Under my dress I was wearing a black satin corset and black seamed stockings teamed with black court shoes. Max and I had had long email exchanges about what I liked to wear and how he liked his submissive to dress. We'd exchanged dozen of photographs of outfits. Before today's meeting Max had asked me to send him pictures of my favourite lingerie and a selection of dresses – without me in them – so that he could choose what I wore for our first real encounter.

From now on whenever we were together, he explained, he would decide what I wore. He would email me instructions and would also go through my wardrobe, and we would go shopping for anything he felt I lacked. And from now on when we were together I wasn't to wear any underwear.

I'd stared at him. Seriously?

Max had nodded.

I hadn't gone braless since God knows when, and I certainly had never gone knickerless. When I protested about how awful fitted clothes looked without some sort of support under them, Max conceded that with some outfits, yes, I could wear a bra, but he would decide which ones, and the only bras I could wear in his company should fasten at the front unless otherwise instructed. A submissive's body no longer belongs to her, he said, and she should always be available for her Master. I stared at him. 'Available?'

He nodded.

Now Max trailed a finger across my shoulders in the same way you might stroke a piece of sculpture. It was the most astonishing sensation, hard to put into words. Dressed to please, elevated to an object of pure desire and pleasure, I have never felt more female or, perversely, more powerful.

'You look fabulous,' Max murmured after a few moments more. 'Put your hands behind your back.'

I did as I was told, lulled by his voice and a peculiar sense of euphoria.

Max caressed my shoulders and neck, his touch proprietorial. One hand stroked up and down my back while the other hand worked its way into the top of my corset, his long, strong fingers cupping one of my breasts. His thumb brushed across my nipple, which stiffened in response. He let out a soft sigh that made me quiver, my skin tingling, electrified by his touch. His hands were cool and almost dispassionate, caressing, squeezing, exploring and kneading.

I gasped as the intensity increased and he nipped and twisted my nipples, before folding the top of the corset down so that first one and then both breasts were exposed.

I could feel the cool air on my naked flesh and a charge of expectation. I could sense his growing excitement along with my own. All the joking and banter were over and I realized that Max wanted and needed this as much as I did. He moved so that he was standing in front of me. I felt his lips close around my nipple, sucking, nipping, biting, drawing my nipple deep into his mouth, making me gasp, the sensations coursing through me like ripples of white light.

As Max pulled away, my body clamoured for more. His lips moved to the other nipple, eagerly licking and sucking his fingers as they worked on the heavy swell of my breasts. As he pulled away, I heard a sound I didn't immediately recognize. An instant later I felt the unexpected bite of something cold and metallic clamping tightly down onto my nipple. I shrieked in surprise and pain, trying to pull away as little teeth bit down harder, holding the clamp fast, and as I exhaled I heard the tinkle of bells.

I discovered later that they were nipple clamps with a string of tiny silver bells hanging from them.

Now every movement, every shudder and every gasp were echoed in silvery tinkling sounds. The teeth bit into my engorged nipples, sending tiny hot splinters of pain and pleasure through me.

'Beautiful,' Max whispered, stroking the bells' strings, making me gasp.

Max and I had talked a lot about what I liked sexually, areas I wanted to explore, things that were a definite no-no and represented a deal breaker – the hard limits beyond which I wouldn't go – and those things that I might like to try once my confidence had grown. I'd told him things I had never told anyone else. I'd just signed off on it, hadn't I? We'd definitely talked about the fact I didn't want to be tied up until I knew Max better, so I didn't think twice when something cool and smooth clicked onto one wrist, although I had a blinding flash of revelation as the second cuff snapped home.

I gasped and opened my mouth to protest. Bugger the no talking rule.

'What the hell do you think you are you doing?' I gasped, little bells tinkling furiously. I struggled to free my hands, even though I knew it was pointless.

'That's what the hell do you think you're doing, *Sir*,' said Max. 'You said no ropes. And now I'm going to have to punish you for talking without permission too.'

I was stunned. Semantics: Max had got me handcuffed and helpless with semantics. There was some part of me that loved the fact that he had outwitted me and another part that was furious. Not much of me was anxious.

'Do you want me to stop?' Max asked, serious now. 'If you're not happy I can always take them off.'

I found it hard to speak.

'Are you OK?' he repeated, seeking an answer. 'I'm not going on until you tell me.'

'Yes, I'm fine, just bloody annoyed,' I snapped, after a second or two, and added more haltingly, 'Sir.'

Max laughed. 'Pleased to hear it,' he said, 'and I'm glad to see you're getting to grips with the Sir thing.' As he spoke he traced the line of my jaw with a finger.

Despite the trick, I felt more excited than I had in years. I also had no doubt that had I asked Max he would have taken the cuffs off. I couldn't have gone this far if I didn't have an underlying trust in him and feel inherently safe. No one else can make that call for you. I trusted him.

'Are you ready?' he said.

Ready for what? 'I think so, yes – Sir,' I said.

'Good,' Max said, and I could hear the warmth and approval in his voice. He led me across the room and had me stand while he settled himself on a chair. He stroked me gently until I was completely still and those little bells finally stopped ringing.

'I'm going to put you across my knee and then I'm going to spank you. But before I do, I want you to ask me to do it,' he said.

I froze. 'I have to *ask*?' I said incredulously.

Max laughed. 'Yes, and you've broken the no talking rule again – and not calling me Sir. You're only supposed to speak when you're spoken to, and only answer the question you've been asked.'

'I'm going to find that hard.'

'Really?' he said, with mock surprise. 'Now ask me.'

I'd never found it particularly easy to ask for what I wanted sexually. Had I told him that? I tried to remember. *Ask?* In my fantasies all this happened without a word being spoken.

'Well?' pressed Max.

'I want you to spank me.'

'*Want?*' There was more than a hint of rebuke; submissives can't demand anything. 'Ask nicely, Sarah.'

It was the kind of thing adults said to small children and said in almost exactly the same tone. A little charge of humiliation stoked the fire of desire.

'Please will you spank me?'

'Better, but not quite good enough. *Sir,*' added Max. 'Ask me again, properly this time.'

'Please will you spank me, Sir?' I murmured, squirming with embarrassment.

'Very good. Here, let me help you.' Very gently he guided me down over his knees, which was not elegant and certainly not easy in handcuffs, with the little clamps biting into my skin and sending little flares, bright as stars, through my consciousness. When you are blindfolded, pain and pleasure are not just sensations but colours; bright, unexpected flashes of colour.

Then, when I was calm, the bells were still and my breathing had slowed, he pulled down my knickers. I was so stunned that I almost stood up again. I had to remind myself that I'd agreed to all this. I had, I really had.

'Gently, gently,' he murmured.

Gently, my arse, I thought, although under the circumstances maybe that wasn't quite the right phrase. I was flooded with a wave of panic and a horrible squirming embarrassment. In my fantasies I was altogether more lithe and the scene of my spanking more subtly lit; certainly I was not in broad daylight in my sitting room. Had Max been expecting lithe? Did Doms get put off? In fantasies they didn't, but in the flesh – the acres of flesh, offered my brain helpfully – maybe they did. I could feel myself blushing scarlet. Then I wondered if it was this, the sense of discomfort and humiliation, that Doms got off on? More than that, this felt like my fantasy – the sense of exposure, the vulnerability. I shivered. I was doing it; this was it.

Max, meanwhile, didn't seem at all put off – quite the reverse, in fact. He made soothing appreciative noises and stroked my thighs and backside, easing the tension from my body, and gradually, remarkably, unexpectedly, I began to relax.

'Gently,' he murmured. 'You're fine, Sarah. Just fine.'

And just when I had been lulled into stillness, Max hit me, one big flat-handed, stinging, spanking slap that ricocheted through my body. The slap wasn't hard, but it was enough to make me cry out in surprise and pain – my whole body flexed.

I had been so busy thinking about the fantasy and more recently thinking about the indignity of having my bum up in the air that it hadn't really occurred to me that spanking would hurt – and it really did hurt. How come I hadn't factored that into my fantasy?

Then Max slapped me again, slightly harder this time, which sent another hot stinging wave coursing through me. Before I could recover, there was another slap and then another.

Instinctively I squealed and kicked, bucking and writhing against his thighs, wanting him to stop, begging him to stop, yet at the same time wanting him to continue. This was what I had dreamt of, this was what I had wanted, and now it was happening I wasn't altogether sure that I liked it. It made me squeal and wriggle and gasp for breath, and I kicked some more as my eyes filled with tears. The bells kept on tinkling, more frantically now.

'If you want me to stop, all you have to do is say the word,' said Max.

I knew that. I really truly knew that. I could make it stop, so why didn't I? Because in among the pain there was something else: a glow of need and desire, a rolling, aching want.

Max slapped me again. Being spanked hurt more than I had ever imagined; it wasn't at all like my fantasy. Yet there was something else lurking under the surface. It was liberating to make a fuss, to be so directly connected to how I felt and to react to it. I'm rationalizing this after the event. At the time it felt like a great raw emotional force steaming through me, and it set me free.

One of the things Max had said to me over lunch was that there was no going back – once you crossed over, there was no unknowing what you discovered about yourself – and I had a glimpse of what he meant. How could anyone sane like something that hurt them? It was impossible to make sense of it, yet it was an amazing, free-fall cascade of sensations with no walls between what I felt and what I was and my reaction to it; it felt as though I was completely connected to every part of myself.

The blows weren't that hard but they were shocking. I gasped for breath, tears trickling down my face, and then between strokes Max began to massage the hot, stinging flesh of my backside, stroking the hand prints, and slowly started to go further, opening my legs wider – touching me, exploring. Letting go and letting him touch me without boundaries, without hindrance, added to my excitement.

I groaned with pure animal pleasure as he found the warm wet folds of my sex and I felt my whole body start to respond as he stroked me in altogether more intimate ways. The pain had brought me so far, and the pleasure that took over was intense and all the deeper for the spanking. I could feel my heart rate quicken, the warm glow across my backside echoing the one that was beginning to grow low down, deep in my belly.

Max slid a finger inside me, making me moan with pleasure. He slid deeper, deliberately brushing my clitoris as his fingers began to work in and out. I was stunned by how intense the sensations were, as if the pain had amplified what I was feeling. Where did the desire come from? Was this about the pain, the embarrassment, the sense of helplessness? I had never experienced anything quite so all-consuming before, and as I began to move with his caress I could feel his erection pressing against my torso through his trousers.

My whole body was focused on his touch as I moved instinctively, relishing the attentions of his knowing fingertips, the way he teased me into reaching out for each delicious sensation.

God, this was fabulous and the sweetest of tortures! I was so close to the edge now that I thought I would die, gasping, whimpering with pure undiluted pleasure as he brought me closer and closer to oblivion. I had not expected this. My hips lifted in time to his touch, longing for release …

'Please,' I whispered, shocked at my own need. 'Please.'

Max chuckled.

Hadn't we just agreed that there would be no sex, not today, perhaps not ever? This was down to me. There was a part of me that had been thinking I could have a 'real' relationship alongside a BDSM one – naïve but true. In an early conversation Max had pointed out that it was quite possible to have a BDSM relationship and never have full sex or in fact any sexual contact.

Never? I'd asked. Never, he'd said. Other couples did it where one was involved with a partner who didn't engage in BDSM.

It had all sounded so perfectly feasible when I'd got my clothes on and we'd been deciding whether to have the sea bass or the lamb for lunch. I had taken everything Max had said to heart, and fondly imagined going off to see someone like Max for a weekly spanking and a bit of light bondage, alongside another more conventional relation-ship, a bit like going to a t'ai chi class or having my legs waxed. I realized now that for me that would be close to impossible. I was aching for him.

'Please,' I sobbed. 'Please.'

'Not yet,' he said. 'And that's the fourth time you've broken the rules.'

'Please, Sir,' I gasped.

How could you feel like this, share this intimacy, this exposure with someone, and then go home to a boyfriend or a husband, girlfriend or wife? I realized I couldn't switch off my emotions and isolate my sexual need; I needed to have both together in the same relationship.

My body was aching for Max in a great rush of animal lust – something that in all the years I'd been having sex, even lust-driven hungry sex, I don't think I'd ever felt before. It was earthier and more physical than anything I had ever experienced. And I could sense Max's excitement growing along with my own. I heard his breath quicken to match mine. Maybe this was where mutual desire overturned the rules?

Eagerly I leaned into his caress. I brushed myself against his engorged cock. It felt like a challenge. Maybe I could make him break the rules. How hard could it be? I was an instant away from the long, tumbling descent towards orgasm. I wanted him to take me there. I wanted to take him with me.

I arched my back. I pressed down onto his lap, brushing myself against his fingertips, seeking his caress, gasping as he stroked my clitoris, riding the great waves that threatened to drown me. I groaned, feeling the first ripples – which was exactly the moment Max stopped.

I howled in protest.

Max laughed and let me slide gently onto the floor.

'I said not yet,' he said, in answer to my indignation and frustration.

'Not yet?' I gasped, ragged, hot and desperate.

'It's your own fault. You can't stick to the rules. No talking. And here, with me, I'm the Dom and things happen according to my timetable, not yours.'

'Are you planning to punish me some more, Sir?' I said, thinking about how much I'd enjoyed my punishment up until now.

'Possibly. By stopping now and going home if you can't be quiet.' He knelt down beside me and unlocked my handcuffs, gently massaging each wrist in turn before taking off my mask. I blinked in the light and peered up at him. His eyes were alight with mischief and delight. I suspected mine were ringed with mascara.

'How are you feeling? Are you OK?'

'Yes, Sir,' I said. He was right: it was getting easier.

'Good. Would you like to touch yourself?'

My eyes widened. *No, I would not.*

'Well, would you?' he repeated.

I'd never admitted to anyone that I masturbated. Not that it had ever come up much in conversation. God, what if he asked me to do it in front of him? I said nothing but my face obviously gave me away.

'I'll take that as a yes,' he said. 'From now on I forbid you to masturbate unless I give you express permission.'

I bristled. 'Are you serious?'

'You are going to be such a pleasure to train,' said Max, laughing. 'I'm making a note of every time you break the rules, you know. And you will pay for every last one you break.'

'Really?' I said.

'Yes, really. And that, in case you hadn't noticed, is another one.'

He helped me to my feet, and as he did he kneaded the tender muscles of my backside, making me wince and momentarily forget the warm, dull, throbbing ache between my legs. Finally he removed the nipple clamps, which made me yelp with pain and then gasp as the blood flooded back into the sensitive flesh. Then he rubbed them, which I thought was a kindness until I realized that actually it made the discomfort much, much worse.

'While we're playing I want you to keep your eyes down and your hands behind your back, as a sign of humility and submission. And now I'd like a cup of tea. Earl Grey. Black.'

I stared at him. My legs were jelly, my whole body was tingling, I'd been a nanosecond from orgasm and the man wanted *tea*?

'Be careful,' he said. Obviously the disbelief showed on my face. 'Remember, humility and submission. Do you have lemon?'

I managed not to swear. Frustrated and annoyed, I teetered into the kitchen and made Max a pot of tea, on a tray with a bone-china cup and saucer, retrieved from a box of nonsense that hadn't seen the light of day for years. I was being sarcastic. If he noticed, he didn't say anything.

'Very nice,' he said, as I slid the tray onto a little table alongside the sofa.

'I'm fresh out of doilies,' I said.

'Next time,' he said, pouring himself a cup. 'And by the way that's another two for the punishment list. Sir and no speaking, remember? When you're not otherwise occupied I would like you to kneel beside me.'

'Kneel?'

He nodded. 'Assuming you want to continue with your training? Or have you changed your mind?'

I could hear from his tone that he was serious. I knelt.

'Would you like to hear about how I got into BDSM?' he asked, setting the cup and saucer back on the side table.

What I wanted was for him to finish what he had started, but I could hardly say that, so instead I said, 'Yes, Sir.'

'Is the right answer,' he said.

Chapter Six

'Nature, who for the perfect maintenance of the
laws of her general equilibrium, has sometimes
need of vices and sometimes of virtues, inspires
now this impulse, now that one, in accordance
with what she requires.'

Marquis de Sade

'I was probably twenty, maybe twenty-one, and my
company had sent me to work in one of their European
offices,' said Max. 'I was green as grass. Anyway, I started
seeing this girl, Eva. A mate of mine set me up with her;
she was a bit older than me, but not much, twenty-three,
twenty-four. Really tiny, attractive.' Max smiled.

'Eva was nothing like any of the girls I'd gone out with
before. She liked a drink, and dancing – and she loved sex.
I'd come from a small town in the south-east, where nice
girls just didn't, so that was one big difference. I couldn't
believe my luck.

'We'd meet up after work – she'd got a little flat near
the railway station. We'd do the usual stuff: there were a
couple of bars, nightclubs, we'd have a few beers, go dancing, drinking, go back to her place.

'Her flat was on the top floor above a row of shops; it was one big room with a shower and toilet off the stairs, all the usual stuff, but the first thing you noticed when you went in was a huge carved four-poster bed.

'God knows where it came from or how old it was. Eva told me it had been there when she moved in. The only way her landlord would have been able to get it downstairs would have been to saw it into pieces, so she told him to leave it. We used to camp out on it, use it as a sofa, as a picnic table, somewhere to watch TV from. Sex, fun, music ...

'Her flat was above a delicatessen. She was so *foreign.*'

'And exciting?' I said.

Max nodded. 'Total culture shock. Anyway, we'd been seeing each other for a couple of months. My best mate, Charlie, was dating Eva's best friend, Greta. We'd all got the weekend off and we'd been planning to do something all together, but at the last minute Greta got called in to work and Charlie said he didn't want to play gooseberry, so there was just Eva and me.

'When I met her at the bus stop she said that there was somewhere she wanted to take me. I didn't really mind where we went as long as I was with her and we ended up back at her place.'

Max smiled. 'She was built like a boy, with short, spiky, white-blonde hair, long skinny legs and the biggest greenest eyes you've ever seen. And she was dynamite between the sheets. She was the most uninhibited person I'd ever met – not that I had been out with that many in my short romantic career. Eva was always up for it, full on, all the time, as far as I could make out.

'She was incredibly vocal, liked to bite and was bossy. Very bossy. I'd never come across anyone like her before. I'd be in bed with her and she would tell me what she wanted: "Hold my hands down, tighter – now fuck me faster, *faster*. That's it and touch me there – just there ..." If I didn't do it right she'd take my hands and show me exactly what it was she wanted, and when she didn't get it she was only too happy to do it herself.

'Up until then the only sex I'd ever had was fumbling around in the dark in the back of a car or in the sports pavilion. Just getting it was enough without thinking about technique.'

Max laughed. 'I've got this memory of her, naked except for leather riding boots and bright red lipstick, showing me *exactly* how she liked to be stroked. I couldn't keep my hands off her. I'm amazed we didn't get ourselves arrested, some of things we got up to.

'She used to tell me I was too British, too uptight; she was probably right.

'I'd been seeing someone back home called Nola. I wasn't that serious about our relationship, but I knew she was. We'd known each other since we were at primary school. Everyone, including our families, was expecting that eventually we'd settle down and get married. She was as steady as a rock, Nola, and she wanted us to get engaged and save up for a house. She used to write to me every week, telling me all about her job in Boots and how all the family were doing.

'Nola was the kind of girl that good boys want to settle down with. She drew the line at French kissing and a bit of heavy petting. Her mum and dad were really strict and she was the same: she thought that nice girls didn't have sex before marriage and barely tolerated it afterwards. She thought that we should wait until we were married before going "the whole way", whereas Eva could barely wait until we got out of the bus station.'

Max laughed again and shook his head. 'So anyway one weekend, I'd got it into my head we were going to have a few beers and head back to Eva's flat, but she'd got other plans. She said that she had a place she wanted to show me. Her English was really good, and she had a funny gravelly voice, and I was totally smitten: I'd have followed her anywhere – anything to keep her sweet. After all, we'd got the whole weekend and I didn't want her getting mad with me.'

Max grinned at me. 'And so we headed to a bar in the town centre where we had gone the first time we met. I remember saying, "Is this it? We've been here before ..."

'Eva shook her head. "No, of course it isn't. Be patient," she said.

'So we got a table and ordered. Apparently it was too early to go wherever she wanted to take me. But it felt like something was going on. She seemed off, edgy, distracted and excited, her eyes working the room, wandering around the bar, glancing up at the clock, watching people come and go as if she was waiting for something to happen. It was nerve-racking. I kept wondering what the hell I was getting myself into.

'The beers didn't take the edge off the mood. I kept wondering if I was being set up. There were plenty of stories about honeytraps and guys getting mugged after following some woman down a dark alley, but I kept thinking: if I was going to get rolled, surely they wouldn't have waited two months to do it? Maybe it was something else; maybe Eva was planning to dump me. Maybe she had met someone else.

'I found myself watching the door, watching Eva, watching the people coming in and out of the bar. By the time we left at around eleven I was ready for just about anything. And I wasn't expecting anything good.

'We grabbed a cab and headed across town. The taxi dropped us at the bottom of the steps that went down into an alley, and it was packed, buzzing with people all on a Friday night out. There were bars and nightclubs with people spilling out of the open doorways; we had to squeeze our way between them.

'I was hanging back, waiting for whatever it was to kick off, till Eva got hold of my arm and pushed her way through. We made our way down the alley to a club. Bouncers look much the same the world over, and there were two big guys in standard dark jeans and leather jackets on the door. As we walked up to them, one of them grinned and touched his cap, and Eva saluted.

'I asked how they knew her. She said she was a regular and that it was one of her favourite places and that she worked there sometimes.

'I asked her why we hadn't gone there before and she just grinned and said that she had needed to know me a bit better before sharing all her secrets.

'"What secrets?" I asked.

'She giggled and tapped the side of her nose. "Soon," she said, "soon. Relax, it's nothing bad ..."

'Anyhow, we joined the queue. There was no name above the club door, no sign; everything looked normal. The only thing that struck me as odd was that lots of punters in the queue were wearing long coats – it was a warm evening, so that was strange – and a lot of the others were carrying holdalls.

Eva had a maxi coat on but she almost always wore it.

'We got to the front desk and there were two huge middle-aged women on the front desk taking the money. They looked liked drag queens: heavy make-up, low-cut tops, smoking like trains. It was obvious that they knew Eva, and while they were saying their hellos the pair of them kept eyeing me up and down. One of them waved us through.

'Inside there was a little bar off to one side. The whole place was heaving with people. It was like a rabbit warren and I couldn't get my head around why we were there. People were smoking and drinking at the bar. To one side of the entrance was a flight of stairs going up and another going down, and a corridor leading off to God knows where. The corridor was lined with doors. There were people everywhere.

'I'd been to a lot of clubs but this one felt different. I

kept thinking I'd made a big mistake going here on my own, and that I should have waited until Charlie and Greta had been able to come with us.

'But Eva was like, "Relax, it's a good place. Good people. You will like it."

'That wasn't how I felt.

'She took hold of my arm and took me through the bar; I could hear music and I was thinking maybe there was a band. Then we got to another set of double doors. I remember looking down at her and realizing she was trembling, and I wondered what the fuck was going on. I thought maybe she was cold but then she looked up at me, and she was all shiny-eyed and excited. Just before she pushed open the doors, she stretched up on tiptoes and said, "Don't be afraid."

'Talk about freaking you out. Then she pushed open the doors.'

'What did you think was going on?' I asked, hanging on his every word.

Max laughed. 'Truth? I hadn't got a clue. We'd been warned about bomb threats and terrorism – there was lots of bad stuff going on – and because this place hadn't got a name outside I just kept thinking: I'm walking straight into trouble here.

'Anyway, the doors opened. I had no idea what to expect, but it sure as hell wasn't what I saw. The room was full of people in all kinds of costumes. It was like a carnival. The music was really loud, and there were strobe lights and a smoke machine. There were people in leather, feathers, bare-breasted, bare-chested; some were dancing. But it wasn't just the audience that surprised me but what was going on on stage.

'There was a naked blonde woman, built like a dancer, and she was strapped to a frame and being flogged by a huge black guy with a shaved head and dressed as a pirate. Both of them had been covered in oil, or maybe it was sweat, but anyway their bodies glistened under the spotlights, and her whole back was criss-crossed with red welts.

'I didn't know what to say or where to look – I'd never seen anything like it, not even in magazines. I wondered why nobody was helping her – crazy – so my first thought in a bondage club was that someone really ought to rescue the blonde; but my second was that she didn't look like she'd thank me for saving her. In a cage next to the frame was another girl, naked except for a cat mask, who had her wrists chained above her head and who was writhing in time to the music. And I got the impression that she was probably next up on the frame …

'I'd heard rumours about clubs like this. I and a gang of the lads from the office had headed for the red light district for a gander the first couple of weeks after I'd arrived, but I had never imagined finding myself in a place like this.'

Max laughed. 'I was bloody terrified and for some reason I kept thinking about Nola back at home, saving up for her bottom drawer. I didn't know where to look. Some of the audience were watching the show, but everyone was treating it like a regular night out, drinking, eating and dancing, as if this sort of thing was perfectly normal, which for them of course it was.

'There were a handful of people dressed in ordinary clothes, me among them, but the vast majority of them were dressed in costumes, fetish clothes, bondage gear, masks, rubber, leather corsets and waistcoats, breeches and boots, all-in-one latex body suits, some almost naked except for straps and buckles – and that included the staff. It certainly explained the coats and the holdalls. It was like Sodom and Gomorrah.

'I looked across and Eva was watching me, probably I think now in case I made a run for it. She asked me if I was OK. I can't remember what I said but I remember her saying, "You can close your mouth now." Then we found a table and she waved the waitress over and ordered us a couple of beers. I just kept gawping. At a table just inside the door there were a man and woman eating, apparently completely oblivious to the man and naked woman kneeling at their feet. On the table next to us were two girls, one dressed as an angel, the other as a devil, who were kissing. I asked Eva if it was a brothel and she laughed and said no, it was a club.

'"People like to come here to be who they are," she said. "They like to get dressed like this and be like this. It's like a playground for people with particular tastes." Then she paused and there was a moment when she looked at me and I knew what was coming. "For people like me," she said. And then – I'll never forget it – she stood up and started to unbutton her coat. Underneath she was wearing a little dress that buttoned down the front. It was really short, so you could see her stocking tops and suspenders. She was also wearing boots – Eva liked boots.

'And she said, "So you like my new outfit?" with a Cheshire cat grin on her face, and came dancing back towards me.

'I said yes, I think, and then I said, "It's short."

'And she said, "It's meant to be. I have very good legs." And with that she peeled off her coat and started to undo her dress.

I stared at Max. 'And you let her?' I asked.

Max laughed. 'I didn't have much choice. There was no way I could have stopped her. I kept thinking: this can't be happening. I was horrified and shocked and turned on – and God knows what else. I jumped up and went to cover her up with her coat, but she shook her head and pushed me away.

'There was an old guy a couple of tables away who was looking her up and down as she was peeling off her dress, and there was a part of me that wanted to punch him and another part that thought: look all you like – she's mine.

'Under the dress Eva was wearing a leather harness that came round over her breasts, round her waist and her hips. And there was a strap that came up between her legs, with a little padlock on it, like a chastity belt, locking it to a waistband. She looked amazing.

'With a total lack of self-consciousness she rolled up her dress and dropped it into her bag, and at the same time pulled out a collar and lead.

'"Do you want to play?" she whispered, holding the lead out towards me.

'All sorts of things were falling into place: the way she liked to be held down; how physical she was; the way she liked me to fight with her for sex, to pin her to the bed; the way she was constantly pushing the boundaries, trying to provoke a reaction.

'I didn't know what you called what she was, but I could feel myself reacting to it. I kind of understood it and knew that I liked it, and that whatever she was I was the other half of it. If she was the question, then I was the answer.'

I stared at Max. 'You knew?'

He nodded. 'Just the same way that you know. So I sat back, crazily calm, watching this mad crazy girl, and she held the collar and lead out again and said, "You want to play?"

'And this time I took it, because there was nothing else that I wanted more. I'd got a hard-on just looking at her. Then she leaned in close and said, "It will be all right. You and I can do anything you like: you can whip me, you can tie me up, you can make me do exactly what you want. I know that you would like to do that. I know that you want to. I can see it in your eyes. I saw it the first night we met. I will love every minute of it. And so will you. I promise …"

'I was nervous, but she was right – I knew it. She knelt down in front of me, and I fastened the collar around her neck and snapped on the lead.

'Then she told me that she had booked us a private playroom upstairs. "Don't worry, I'll teach you everything you need to know," she said. "You will be the best Master I have ever had."

'I had no idea what that meant, but then she reached up to pull me in close for a kiss.

'I laughed and kissed her back, and as I did she pushed something hard and metallic between my lips. It was a padlock key.

'"You're going to need that," Eva said.'

Chapter Seven

'… the only way to a woman's heart is along the
path of torment. I know none other as sure.'
Marquis de Sade

'So what happened next?' I asked, completely caught up in
Eva and Max's story. I'm nosey, I'm a storyteller. I love the
narrative of other people's lives. I wanted to know how it
turned out and what Eva taught him – although it did
occur to me that the chances were I might find out anyway.
My knees ached from kneeling on the floor beside him,
and I had completely forgotten the rules about not speaking unless spoken to and calling Max 'Sir'. A fact not lost
on him. He offered me his hand.

'What happens next? Next, Sarah, I punish you for
breaking the rules. Stand up.'

I hesitated for an instant and then saw the look on Max's
face. He wasn't joking.

'Pain and pleasure', he said, 'are close companions. Like
opposite sides of the same coin. I'll make sure that when
you're with me you experience both, but sometimes there
will be only pain – remember that. Now stand up and face
the wall. Put your hands flat against the wall, level with
your shoulders.'

I did as I was told. Max stood behind me, and with his foot eased my feet apart until they were at shoulder width. From the corner of my eye I could see him taking something from the leather holdall he had brought with him. Something with a handle, something around two feet long and topped with a head of long suede leather strips.

'This is one of my favourite toys, thanks to Eva,' Max said. 'It's a flogger. She loved being flogged. I have a man who makes them for me.' As Max spoke he drew the narrow strips through his closed fingers and then swished them to and fro thoughtfully. 'How many times do you think you've broken the rules today?' he asked, before trailing the long strands of the flogger down over my shoulders and back, the leather thongs making my skin tingle.

'I don't know – a few …' I grimaced and bit my lip. 'Sir,' I added as an afterthought.

'You see, that's another one. What do you think? Six, eight, maybe twelve times since I arrived?'

'About six, I think, Sir,' I said.

Max laughed. 'Maybe I should add another stroke for lying? We both know that it's closer to twelve. Let's split the difference, shall we? Let's call it ten. I'm going to flog you, Sarah. And I want you to the count the strokes for me.'

I stiffened, but managed to avoid the possibility of earning myself another stroke by – for once – holding my tongue. Max draped the fronds of the flogger over my shoulder again and drew them across my skin, more slowly this time. They were soft, cool, practically a caress. I shivered.

'Feel good?' he said.

'Yes, Sir,' I whispered. They felt like silk. They set my nerves tingling. So good. So very soft. I closed my eyes. In my books I had imagined this moment a hundred times.

'Let go. I won't do anything to you that you don't want or can't cope with, and you always have the safe words – remember that. Let me show you what you're capable of loving ...'

I shivered, lulled by his voice, soft, warm and dark.

'Come with me.' It was an invitation to surrender. Some part of me understood what he wanted but I wasn't sure that I could, or that I was ready. How do you learn to let go and lose yourself in sensation? There was a split second when I was aware of the narrow suede leather strips sliding away and an instant later a stinging, stunning, white-hot crackle of leather across my back. The tails of the flogger wrapped around me so that the very end of the thongs caught my ribs and breast. The feeling took my breath away.

'If you don't count them, then the strokes don't count either,' Max said, as the flogger landed for a second time.

'Two, Sir,' I gasped, every cell, every fibre of my body awakened by the flogger's kiss.

The leather strips found their mark again.

'Three,' I hissed.

The suede thongs that had felt so smooth and so very soft when stroked over my back grazed into my skin like hot fingers. I could hear them moving through the air an instant before feeling them hit home, and between strokes

I could hear Max breathing from the effort of using the flogger, as my skin grew hot and tingled.

I heard the swish of the tails again and closed my eyes.

'Four.' The expectation and the sensation were building with every stroke, a rush of endorphins cascading, intense and all consuming, and blowing away all thoughts; everything was gone but the here and now, the feel of the flogger, the sound of my ragged breathing, the count and the glowing heat of each stroke as it rolled through me.

'Five,' I cried out. Tingling all over now, my skin feeling as if it was glowing red hot, I was gasping, trying hard to retain my control.

'It's all right,' he said. 'Let go. I'm here ...'

'Six.' I am losing myself in pain. All there is is the sound of my voice and the explosive sensation of the flogger, and I know I can call a halt but I don't want to, I don't – and then Max hits me again, leather and heat, crackling, rippling through my nerve endings.

'Seven.' The word is a gasp. I am being sucked under by the flogger's kiss but I'm nearly home now. Just three more strokes ...

'Eight.' The stroke is harder still, I think, but I can't gauge it, I'm so lost inside what I am feeling. I am sobbing for breath and for him to stop, but I don't say the safe words. I feel a great rush of euphoria.

'Nine' – I am almost done.

'Ten,' and my knees buckle and Max is there to catch me.

'Good girl,' he murmurs. 'Good girl.' Now his lips are on my neck and shoulders, scattering feathery kisses that light beacons in my mind. His fingers find my breasts, and he is teasing the nipples, twisting and tugging, and I feel the great surge of desire I felt earlier rekindle. I'm trembling as he guides me to a side table and lifts me up onto it, pressing me down onto the cool solid wood so that my back, red hot, striped and alight with sensations, slides down onto the cold shiny surface.

The chill is a stark contrast to the heat from the welts, but before I can surrender to the coolness Max spreads my legs and stands between them, leaning over me, stroking my shoulders and breasts, touching, nipping, and then kissing, licking and sucking hard my dark stiff nipples.

I arch up towards him as the feelings of pleasure flood through me, hot on the heels of the pain – intense and heady. His fingers are between my legs now and I'm breathing hard as he draws first one nipple and then the other into his mouth; I am wet – his fingers slide into me, his thumb brushing my clitoris.

I am gasping, white hot with need and hunger, and then slowly but relentlessly his tongue follows his fingers. He is kissing and sucking my nipples, pressing his lips to the junction between my breasts, kissing and licking down over my ribs.

He laps at my navel, pressing kisses into my belly, fluttering down to the rise of my sex, opening me up, all the while murmuring softly, whispering words of encouragement and approval, and then his tongue slides down over my clitoris, and I am lost – totally, totally lost.

I cry out in pleasure. He pulls back a little, making me work for his touch. My hips lift to chase his tongue and I am wanton, opening to him. He laps and licks and sucks, taking me higher and higher until I think I might faint. His hands cup my backside, pressing into the handprints from the spanking, pulling me onto his mouth, fucking me with his tongue, lapping at my clitoris, I am moaning and begging – and all at once I am there, and totally, totally consumed. As I tumble over the edge into oblivion I know that Max is right: I will never be the same again.

Chapter Eight

'But seduction isn't making someone do what
they don't want to do. Seduction is enticing
someone into doing what they secretly
want to do already.'
Waiter Rant

When Max finally left I put on a bathrobe, made a pot of
tea and went to sit in the garden. Despite the bright
sunshine I felt shivery and feverish. One of the last things
Max had said as he was leaving was that I should eat something, which made me smile. Of all the words of support
and encouragement I was hoping for, 'You should have a
sandwich' wasn't one of them.

As he slipped on his jacket, he said, 'I'll ring you this
evening. And if you want to talk to me before that then all
you have to do is call. I'll pick up.' He paused and traced
the line of my jaw with his fingertip. 'I'm not going to
play you or make you wait or make you doubt either me
or yourself. You don't have to agonize about what I think
of you, or whether I'll ring you or talk to you, or whether
something wasn't right. It was perfect, beautiful – and
you're beautiful.'

I smiled, and leant into his caress. I felt weepy.

Max leaned in closer and kissed me on the cheek. I shivered.

'Are you OK?'

I nodded, oblivious to the answering-with-words rule. He tipped my face up towards him so that he could look into my eyes. 'Do you want to talk now? I can stay if you want me to.'

'No, I'm fine. Really, truly,' I said, with a shake of the head. It was true. I needed to think about this on my own, not talk it over. 'But you're right. It was a big step.'

He waited.

'And I'm really OK with it. It's what I wanted – what I want,' I said. 'It's just a lot to take in.'

'Do you want me to make you that sandwich?'

I laughed. 'No, really. I'm fine. Please, go. I'll talk to you later.'

'OK.'

Max looked so innocuous as he picked up his leather holdall and made his way to the door. No one would guess what was in it, nor what this tall, distinguished man in his beautifully cut suit had spent the afternoon doing to me.

When he had gone, I started to cry.

I suppose I was in shock. I'd taken a huge first step after a lifetime of anticipation; finally all the things I had fantasized and dreamt about had happened – were happening. Was it good? Yes, better than I could have hoped. Was it as I had imagined? No, it wasn't. Real-life sex and BDSM aren't seamless and wordless, or painless; it's a journey towards finding the things you want and desire, not a destination in itself. And I knew that if I wanted it then this was just the start.

I went into the kitchen and made a sandwich. Max was right – it did make me feel better.

One of the things that make BDSM such a compelling game – and different from the majority of other relationships – is that wherever you are, whatever you're doing, a sub and Dom always share a secret. Whatever appears to be happening on the surface, there is almost always something else going on beneath that surface. It is fun, it builds trust, and it is totally addictive.

After we had met a few times at my place, Max suggested that we go out together rather than just play on home ground. He arranged to come and pick me up from my house, having emailed explicit instructions about what I was to wear for our date.

He'd booked us a table at a fabulous restaurant on the north Norfolk coast. It was under new management and newly refurbished, had been in the Sunday papers and was somewhere I'd been wanting to go to since it had re-opened. I wasn't exactly sure how Max had managed to get us a table on a Friday evening, and I certainly wasn't complaining, but once we actually arrived I wasn't so sure.

As we pulled into the car park Max looked across at me and smiled. 'All ready?'

I raised my eyebrows and pulled a face. I was so nervous that I couldn't speak.

He grinned. 'Trust me,' he said. 'You'll be fine. You wanted to come here, remember. And who wouldn't? I read the reviews.'

I'd like to say that I nodded but I didn't. I couldn't remember a time as an adult when I'd felt so nervous or so excited, and besides I was getting to grips with the rules. No speaking unless I was given permission.

Since that first meeting at my house we had met up three or four times to continue my training. We had spoken dozens of times on the phone, and he would text me at odd times during the day. One of the things I was beginning to appreciate was that whenever we spoke Max was always the same, calm, funny, quick – and nothing I asked him seemed to faze him or wrong-foot him, whether it was about BDSM or about his personal life. It was a quality I really valued and it made trusting him and opening up to him all the easier.

Tonight he looked great. He was wearing a dark suit cut to make the most of his broad shoulders, a crisp white shirt, red tie and cufflinks. He looked gorgeous – distinguished – and smelt wonderful. He was the perfect dinner date: polite, attentive and confident without being pushy or arrogant. People always treated Max as if he was somebody.

He got out of the car first, taking a gift bag from the back seat. Then he came round to my side of the car, opened the car door for me and took my hand. It was a warm evening but I was trembling. He tucked my hand up over his arm. I was a little unsteady in new high heels, so we made slow progress across the gravel. I'd spent hours getting ready for tonight: my hair looked great and my make-up was flawless.

Inside the restaurant it was even warmer. Prime time, Friday evening and the place was jumping. The foyer was full of fresh flowers. There were people in fabulous clothes sitting up at the bar drinking cocktails and laughing. I could hear the muffled hubbub of conversation from the dining room and the sound of cutlery on china. The place was elegant, smart, full. My pulse was pounding in my ears and I had an odd sense of unreality, as if I was walking onto a film set.

Although it was warm I was wearing a classic Burberry trench coat, along with pearl earrings, my high heels and black hold-ups. Other than that – although no one would ever guess it – I was completely naked under my coat.

I glanced across at Max. If you think this was a big ask you wouldn't be wrong, although it had seemed like fun when he'd emailed me my instructions, like a dare – and of course I had had the choice to say no.

Max smiled at me, ignoring my anxious looks as we headed past the bar towards the dining room. He patted my hand as my eyes widened. I had thought we'd at least stop and have a drink, and that at some point during my first white wine spritzer he would rescue me, maybe after a little teasing, but no: at the door to the restaurant he chatted casually to the maître d', his grip tightening just a fraction as I started to panic.

It was barely a moment or two before a waiter came over to show us to our table. It was in the centre of the restaurant and I knew without a shadow of a doubt that Max had asked for it on purpose. He gently guided me towards it, resting his hand in the small of my back. I could feel my panic rising.

The waiter pulled out my chair. 'May I take madam's coat?' he asked, holding out a hand.

I glanced at Max, who smiled wolfishly and indicated with a nod of his head that I should comply.

Time slowed to a crawl. I swear I heard my pulse rate double. I couldn't quite believe what Max was suggesting and I was waiting for him to call a halt. Surely he didn't seriously expect me to take my coat off here? I hesitated and imagined the scene, the humiliation, the chaos, and felt my colour rising.

The waiter waited.

Very slowly I unfastened the top button of my coat, feeling a growing sense of panic. I could feel Max looking at me and looked up. His smile held. Our eyes met; his were full of mischief.

The waiter stepped closer.

My fingers moved down towards the second button. As I was about to undo it Max said, 'Why don't you go and freshen up your lipstick before we eat?' And handed me the gift bag that he had brought in from the car.

I stopped and stared at him. 'Take your time,' he added.

Heart racing, I headed for the ladies' toilets. In the cubicle I took a moment or two to catch my breath before undoing the bag. Inside was my dress, a clingy little sequinned number, a matching pashmina and a tiny clutch bag. I slipped the dress on over my head and shimmied it down over my hips, making an effort to compose myself, and I giggled. Then I giggled some more. All my life I had always been the good girl, the sensible, responsible one, and it felt so good to break out. No harm done – none at all – but what a rush! I couldn't stop smiling.

I also did exactly what Max suggested and took my time before going back out. I washed my hands, tidied my hair, touched up my lipstick and make-up. I couldn't help noticing that you could see my nipples through the thin fabric of my dress and even a pashmina couldn't disguise the way my breasts moved without a bra.

I walked slowly back to the table, trying to suppress the grin. Max watched me every step of the way. He was smiling. In my absence he had ordered the wine.

'You look wonderful,' he said, as I finally settled at the table and he poured me a glass. 'Now, how about we discuss where we go from here? Is there anything you would like to talk about?'

'Besides brinkmanship?' I asked, taking a long pull on my wine.

'Tell me you didn't enjoy it?' he whispered, eyes bright with amusement.

'I'm not sure "enjoy" is the right word. Have you already ordered?'

Max nodded. 'So what would you like to talk about?' he said.

'Eva,' I said, leaning in closer. 'I want to know what happened next. In the night club, after she gave you the key, Sir.'

Max smiled. 'OK. Well, up until I met Eva it had never occurred to me that women really enjoyed sex. Or at least not nice girls.' He grinned. 'What can I say? I grew up in a small village. Anyway, I'd seen some films in a friend's garage when I was a teenager. It was the usual kind of stuff, pretty tame now compared to what you get on the internet. One of them, towards the end of the reel, was of a girl being put over her boyfriend's knee and spanked for damaging his car.

'The other guys I was watching it with were hooting about the car. I assumed the people who made the film must have forced her to do it or paid her and I was embarrassed that it turned me on. It never occurred to me in a million years that she might have enjoyed it too. Not until that first night with Eva at the club.'

Chapter Nine

'It's just human. We all have the jungle inside of
us. We all have wants and needs and desires,
strange as they may seem. If you stop to think
about it, we're all pretty creative, cooking up all
these fantasies. It's like a kind of poetry.'
Diane Frolov and Andrew Schneider

'After she'd given me the key, Eva led me upstairs to a
room she'd booked for us.' Max laughed. 'To be frank, I
didn't know whether to be turned on or terrified. The
place was like a maze; everywhere you looked there were
things I'd never seen before. Upstairs on the first floor they
used to have some communal playrooms. Eva called them
the galleries and you could just walk through them. In the
first one there were two blondes, maybe in their twenties,
with a big tall guy who looked like a rugby player. He was
fucking one and licking the other one's pussy.' Max
grinned. 'They were loving it. And then there was a girl
called Trude, who liked to paint herself all over – naked,
pierced – and some guy giving another guy a blow job on
the stairs. In the back room there was a man suspended
from the ceiling, hog-tied on a huge metal candelabra; he
was gagged, and had weights hanging from his balls. And

right in the middle of the room was a young guy, athletic, probably in his twenties, all rippling oiled muscle, up on all fours on a plinth, being buggered by a man dressed as a bear.'

'Are you serious?' I said.

Max laughed. 'Oh God yes. You've never seen anything like it. It was like the craziest circus ever mixed with the *Kama Sutra*. I didn't know where to look or what to look at next. Eva kept laughing at me; I'd got her on a leash, but it was more a way of ensuring that I didn't get lost than me leading her anywhere. I remember the bear winked at me and Eva said, "Do you want to join them? We can always ask. I'm sure they wouldn't mind." I was stunned.

'Anyway, we got to a room on the next floor and Eva said that there was someone she wanted me to meet. I was just hoping to hell it wasn't the bear man. She pushed the door open. Inside was a woman dressed in leather shorts, peaked cap and bikini top. She was probably in her late twenties or early thirties, hard-looking, with the most amazing muscular body. She was all smiles, and held out a hand. She told me her name was Jessa, that she was a friend of Eva's and that she was going to show me how to train her. I wasn't altogether sure what she meant – Eva seemed pretty well trained to me.

'She laughed and said something like, "Actually, I will be helping to train you. Eva said that you are a natural and that you just need a little instruction."

'I thought that was over-egging the pudding. I was thinking I'd probably need a lot but I didn't let on. It was the first time I saw a real Dom in action.

'Eva was about to say something but Jessa turned round and snapped, "Be quiet. On your knees. Now."

'I was used to orders but not like this.

'Eva did as she was told, her eyes down in submission. Jessa stood in front of her, legs spread, hands on her hips, and said, "Kiss my boots."

'And she did, as though in an act of worship. It looked horny as hell. Jessa explained that what Eva wanted and needed was for me to take control: for her, controlling was part of showing that I cared. Do you understand, Sarah?'

Max looked at me.

I nodded. 'I think so, but weren't you nervous about getting it wrong or hurting her?'

'Yes, but I wanted to be with Eva and I kind of understood. And I could see from her expression that Eva was clearly enjoying it. Then Jessa picked up a length of rope that was over the back of a chair and said, "I'm going to show you how to tie her and beat her, and then we will share her. Is that acceptable?"

'I'm not sure what shocked me the most: beating Eva or sharing her with another woman. When I didn't reply she said, "It will all become perfectly clear."

Then she ordered Eva to stand up and told her to hold out her hands.

'Jessa really liked rope – the way it looked and the marks it left. During the time we were friends she spent hours showing me how to tie someone up, how to ensure you weren't tying them too tightly or cutting off the circulation. She was a great Dom; being with her was like doing Bondage 101, and as she talked she demonstrated on Eva. That night we ended up binding the rope around Eva's wrists in long cuffs, from the wrist to halfway up her forearm.'

Max took my hand and drew his finger up my arm to show me what he meant, as the waiter delivered our first course. Max thanked him and waited till he was out of earshot before saying, 'Just as Jessa was finishing off the knots she said, "Were you ever a Scout?" I couldn't work out if she was taking the mickey or not, but she assured me that she wasn't. Knots are very useful, she said, and I should get a book and practise,' Max said

'Really?' I said, with a grin. 'Are you serious?'

Max nodded. 'Yes, and she bought me one that year for Christmas. I think I've still got it somewhere. Jessa was fabulous, very intense, very serious – just how you would imagine a real Dominatrix to be. She was also a sweetheart, really funny and great company. She and I were friends for years, even after Eva.

'Anyway, the rooms at the club were designed to accommodate all sorts of tastes. There were places to tie your partner in, plastic sheeting, ropes, chains. In the room we were in there was a metal bar secured to the ceiling. Jessa threw a length of rope and tied Eva off so that her hands were above her head. Jessa was all safety, making sure that you could get your sub down in a hurry if need be. She had a set of tools and toys in a canvas roll and used to unpack them like a surgeon before we started to play, and she always had a pair of scissors or a knife handy in a pouch on her belt.

'Once we'd got Eva secured to the bar she handed me an adjustable pole with bolt hooks at either end and a pair of cuffs to put round Eva's ankles in order to spread her legs. I was shaking so much I could barely undo the buckles.'

He looked at me across the table. I'd barely touched my starter.

'Have you ever seen *The Sorcerer's Apprentice*?' Max said with a grin as he made a start on his pâté. 'That was me, handing Jessa lengths of ropes and pieces of equipment. But when I looked up at Eva, she grinned and blew me a kiss. I knew she was enjoying it and I knew she was right: this was me. It just felt right. Then Jessa took a cloth from the pocket of her shorts and gagged Eva.

'You don't gag someone unless you know them really well, so that you can spot if there is anything wrong. You don't want them to choke. I always use a ball gag – they are safer. Jess tied the knot tightly, pulling the fabric so that it sat between Eva's lips. Once it was in place she grabbed hold of Eva's chin and licked her cheek. She told her how gorgeous she was and how glad she was that she had invited her to come and play with us.

'It felt like I was watching a film. Jess took a thinner cord from the chair and bound Eva's breasts – it was the first time I'd ever seen breast bondage.'

I stared at him, feeling my jaw drop. Although Max was speaking in hushed tones, it felt extraordinary to be having this kind of conversation in such a public place. I looked round. No one else seemed to be taking a blind bit of notice. I wondered what they were all talking about; my best bet was that it wasn't breast bondage.

He grinned. 'Jessa caught hold of one of her nipples and pulled her breast away from her ribs. Eva really yelped and for a split second I thought about stepping in and stopping her. That was until I saw the expression on her face. She tipped her head back and let out a long throaty moan while Jessa wrapped the cord tightly round her breast – and I mean really tightly. Then Jessa bent down and sucked her nipples.'

I made an effort to close my mouth. 'Does it hurt?'

'It makes the flesh swell and the nipple very full and very sensitive – you'll like it,' he said, watching my face. 'So then Jessa handed me the cord. I was all fingers and thumbs, not helped by Eva wriggling and purring or by me having a raging hard-on. In the end Jessa had to help. She grabbed hold of Eva and pulled her breast out harder than I could possibly have done and said, "Tie it now. Tie it tight. As close to the place where the skin meets her chest as you can." So I did as I was told, badly. It was nowhere near tight enough, so she made me do it again, and it slipped off again. It has to be tight enough to hold but not so tight that it restricts too many of the blood vessels. Finally I got it. Then she bent down and sucked Eva's nipple into her mouth. And I sucked the other one.'

Max's voice was low now and intimate, and I felt my body responding to his story.

'It was incredible. I could see Jessa and feel Eva moving, smell her: she was hot and I was so turned on. Between them Eva and Jessa were great teachers and helped me to understand and enjoy what was already there. I learnt fast. Once I'd got Eva settled Jessa took me over to her roll of toys, which she'd laid out on a dresser, and told me to choose whatever I liked. There were canes and whips, short floggers, a riding crop, clamps, ropes, clothes pegs, a ball gag, handcuffs and a dildo in a harness that I guessed was for Jessa. I just stood and stared. I couldn't think much beyond fucking Eva. Jessa said that sex was always there and was the easy option, but that she planned to beat her first and make her earn her reward.

'So she picked up a very thin, very flexible cane, which she bent into a curve. And she said, "Eva doesn't like this, not at all." The curve almost matched the grin on her face.

'I wasn't quite sure I understood. I remember asking if she was going to use it on Eva even though she didn't like it and Jessa shook her head. "Sadly not. You rapidly discover the things that your submissive enjoys. You need to talk about what you like and find a common ground. It doesn't mean you can't push it a little – experiment together – but if you want them to keep playing and scratching your itch you have to take them a little at a time, gently, gently, training them to like what you like and vice versa. It's not something you can rush." She sighed, bending the cane one more time, and then put it down. 'And sadly sometimes you have to give up. You don't want them to walk away, do you?'

'I asked her what Eva liked, and as I did it occurred to me that we were talking about her as if she wasn't there. Jessa started picking up things from her pack to show me.

'"The crop, the driving whip and the flogger ..." She ran through a list and explained that Eva was not so much into pain as into submission – being made to do things, being made to feel vulnerable. She liked her hair being pulled and insertion – things being put into her. She liked to be naked when everyone else was dressed. She was also bi, which I hadn't known.'

I realized that while Max has been talking, I had eaten my starter and hadn't tasted a mouthful. The joke wasn't lost on me: all the time I'd waited to come here for the food and now I was here I wasn't remotely interested in it. As soon as the plates were cleared and the main course served Max refilled my glass and resumed his story.

'Jessa taught me a lot: that you build the pain up slowly – a sub can often take more if you start gently and build up the intensity with each stroke. And always to agree a safe word.'

Max turned his attention to his meal.

'Aren't you afraid that by telling me all this you're going to expose all your secrets and spoil it?' I asked.

Max shrugged. 'You wanted to know. And I'm telling you because I know you want to hear – and I know you want to feel it.'

I stared at him.

He smiled. 'Don't you?' he said. 'And you seem to have forgotten the no talking unless spoken to rule.' Then, leaning in closer as if to kiss me gently on my cheek, he whispered in my ear, his hand brushing my breast. I shivered. 'Imagine them bound and clamped,' he said. 'It seems like a suitable punishment.'

I swallowed hard and he grinned.

'Anyway, Jessa picked up the cane and stroked Eva's breasts with it. Eva tried to pull away. Jessa drew the cane across Eva's breasts and very gently tapped them. She had already told me that you sometimes need to push the boundaries. Eva was wide-eyed, eyes flashing. Jessa liked to tease and flicked Eva's breasts with the cane. Then she flicked them again, this time with a sharp, snappy little strike, and Eva squealed through her gag. I was torn between rescuing her and enjoying what I was watching.

'Then Jessa tapped the padlock that fastened the strap between Eva's legs and asked me if I had the key.

'I knew that I had and patted my pockets, not sure in the heat of the moment what I'd done with it. But I found it, pulled it out and offered it to Jessa, who shook her head and said, "She's yours, not mine. You should do it." And as she spoke she dropped the cane back onto the table and picked up a flogger.'

Max laughed and shook his head. 'I was a mess. I was there for ages. I couldn't get the key into the lock. My fingers shook, and I could feel heat coming from Eva's body and smell the scent of her mingled with the leather. In the end I knelt down and finally undid the strap. Then I couldn't help myself: I kissed her, licking her sex with my tongue. She was so wet, so ready. At which point Jessa – all business – tapped me on the shoulder and said, "Later," and handed me the flogger.

'I'm not sure that I was that keen to wait, but then she showed me how to hit and where to hit – avoiding the kidneys and the sciatic nerve; and how to begin slowly and how to build it up, stroke by stroke. And with each stroke it felt more and more as though I was coming home. It felt good – really good.

'After twelve strokes, we untied Eva and let her down. She sank to her knees, pressing her lips to Jessa's feet and then to her pussy. Jessa gave Eva permission. Eva unfastened the snaps at either side of Jessa's shorts and peeled them away. Underneath Jessa was shaved. It was the first time I'd seen a grown woman like that – you could see the slit and the bud of her clitoris peeking out. Jessa settled herself back on the bed with Eva on all fours between her legs, lapping and sucking her. It was the sexiest thing I'd ever seen; I'd never seen anything so horny in my life. I kept wondering just how much longer I could hold it together without coming.

'Then Jessa beckoned me over and invited me to join in. "Time to enjoy her," she said, all the while Eva was licking her. Then Jessa threw back her head, locking her fingers in Eva's hair, and just let go.

'I didn't need telling twice. I stripped off and sank into Eva. There was no way I was going to last for long – I kept trying to hold back but it was pointless. She was trying to tip me over the edge. I felt her fingers brushing my balls as she started to rub her clit – she was still tonguing Jessa, while her pussy was clutching tightly at my cock. I closed my eyes, desperately trying to hang on, trying to make it last, but it was a lost cause. I totally lost it: I drove into her, wild, desperate, and that was it. Totally spent, I collapsed onto the bed and then rolled over onto my back, completely and utterly shot.

'I woke between the two of them God knows how much later, an arm round each. Jessa was sound asleep but my waking up woke Eva. She opened her eyes and before I could say anything she was on her knees, creeping down over my chest and taking me in her mouth – and I couldn't help myself. It was a long, long night.'

I stared at him.

Max grinned. 'Satisfied?'

I nodded.

He beckoned me closer.

'Eat up. There is a price for all this curiosity,' he said, eyes bright.

Chapter Ten

'Sexual pleasure in woman is a kind of magic spell;
it demands complete abandon.'

Simone de Beauvoir

'So how's the new man working out, then?' asked Gabbie, forking a great pile of lasagne into her open mouth. It was a girls'-get-together night. A lot of wine had been consumed and there were puddings on standby in the fridge.

Helen, who was currently sitting on the other side of the table, wiped something tomato-ey off her chin and rolled her eyes. 'You mean Rob? He's OK, but he's a bit wet, to be honest. I really want someone with a bit more life in him. You know, a bit more ...' She made a noise and a gesture that implied vigour.

We all raised our eyebrows in unison. There is an unofficial credo in our gang: *We've all come too far to settle for a poor compromise.* Almost every time the four of us get together, at least one of us says it about something. Helen, not needing to be told, held up her hands in surrender. 'I know, I know,' she said. 'He has to go, but not until after we get back from Crete.'

'You're going on holiday with him?' asked Gabbie, incredulously.

'Why not? He invited me, and besides I could do with a bit of sunshine. His sister has got a place out there. A villa, I think.'

'Oh God, don't tell me,' sighed Gabbie, slapping her hand to her forehead. 'He and the family used to go out there every summer before he got divorced.'

'Stop it,' said Helen, flicking a piece of lettuce at her.

'Maybe he'll redeem himself,' said Joan, more kindly.

'We did warn you,' said Gabbie. 'Rob didn't strike me as someone with a whole lot of oomph.'

'I know, but to be fair I think you made him nervous, Gabbie.'

Gabbie pulled an 'as if' face.

'He was expecting to come for a walk on the beach with the dogs and a few friends, not to be cross-examined by experts,' said Helen. 'You frightened him.'

Gabbie laughed. 'He needs to grow a pair.'

'How about you, Sarah?' Helen asked, trying to move herself out of the spotlight. 'How's the manhunt coming along?' They all knew that I was internet dating and had been seeing a few people, although none of them knew what sort of sites I'd signed up for.

Before I could reply, Joan, talking with her mouth full, waved her hands around and said, 'Hang on. I knew there was something I meant to tell you. I've found *the* most perfect man for Sarah.'

Everyone looked at her. 'Oh no, you didn't meet him at church, did you? He's not a God botherer, is he?' asked Gabbie.

'No,' said Joan, looking wounded.

'Or another writer?' asked Helen.

'No, he makes bespoke kitchens,' said Joan. 'Really beautiful – top end, gorgeous.'

Around the table everyone nodded enthusiastically. Good with his hands, practical, creative – I could see the three of them stacking up the plus points before they'd even clapped eyes on the man.

I started to speak but no one was paying a blind bit of attention to me.

'And he comes highly recommended,' Joan continued. She didn't expand on whether that was kitchen or relationship related. Joan managed a cookshop that stocks the most amazingly expensive gadgets and has a deli and wine section. Kitchen designers and fitters were part of her world.

'And how were you planning to get him to meet Sarah?' asked Helen.

'Divine intervention,' laughed Gabbie, taking a long sip of her wine.

'Or we could all hang around in the deli section and drive him on to her – you know, like sheep-dogs,' Helen suggested.

Joan puffed out her cheeks. She was indignant: she was trying to be helpful. Joan is lovely; she is always kind and good, and really pretty in a wholesome way. Her stupid husband had left her for a twenty-three-year-old girl who worked in their local garage, who broke his heart and took his money, and then he had been furious with Joan when she wouldn't take him back.

'Don't be ridiculous,' Joan said. 'We're having an open evening at the barn at the beginning of next month. I've already invited Shaun and I was thinking you could all come along. He's in Tuscany at the moment, fitting a friend's kitchen.'

Everyone nodded; I think the Tuscany thing clinched it.

'So promotional evening it is, then,' said Helen, refilling her glass. 'Here's to Shaun.'

'Oh yes, *Shaun*, right. And Helen can get shit-faced on the cocktails again,' hooted Gabbie. Everyone was off again. One bad thing about having good girl friends is that they all have memories like elephants: nothing is ever forgotten.

'That was a long time ago,' protested Helen. 'And I was on tablets. And you're one to talk. What about the time –'

'Anyway,' said Joan, dragging the conversation back on track, 'what I'm saying is that Shaun is really lovely, he loves cooking, he's divorced and he wears nice clothes.'

'And he has friends in Tuscany,' said Gabbie.

'Gay?' suggested Helen.

'No. No, he's not,' said Joan. 'I asked him.'

I hated to spoil their fun ...

'You asked him if he was gay?' said Gabbie. 'Really?'

'We got talking. He doesn't know many people round here,' said Joan.

'I'd like to have been there to hear that conversation,' said Gabbie.

'And I've already told him about Sarah. He seemed quite keen.'

... but I was going to have to.

'You did?' I said, finally managing to get a word in. 'What have you told him, Joan?'

'He's not seeing anyone at the moment. And he's hunky and hairy –'

'*What did you tell him?*'

'Maybe you should save him for yourself?' suggested Helen, sucking the sour cream off another potato wedge.

Joan shook her head. Her moving on from a bad break-up involved a complex, and from what I could make out, rather one-sided relationship with God, and two fox terriers. 'No, he's not my type, but as soon as I saw him I thought he would be perfect for Sarah,' said Joan. 'Just perfect.'

'In that case we should *all* go to Joan's next do,' suggested Gabbie. 'When is it?'

'Tenth of next month,' offered Joan. 'What is that – five, six weeks?'

Gabbie pulled a face. 'Oh, that's too long. Maybe you should just give him Sarah's number. I mean, why wait? Or is he in Tuscany for six weeks?'

In the end I held up my hands to stop the clamour and shouted, 'Stop.' I hadn't got any plans to tell them about Max, and maybe I should have carried on with the plan, but I didn't want Joan fixing me up with someone, and certainly not giving him my phone number, so I said, 'Actually, I'm already seeing someone.'

Talk about stopping the party dead. All three of them swung round to stare at me.

'I thought you were going to give up on men after Henry?' said Helen.

'Are you just *saying* that you've met someone?' said Joan.

'No, I'm a bit old for an imaginary boyfriend. I've been seeing him for a few weeks now. Anyway you know I've been seeing people, Joan: you're my safe call.'

'Well, I know. I just thought you'd gone off the boil a bit lately.'

'So what's he like, then?' asked Gabbie.

I didn't know where to start.

'Oh, come on, Sarah, spill the beans. It's not like you to keep a secret,' pressed Gabbie.

She was right. It wasn't. I am notorious for telling everyone everything. I've shamelessly robbed my private life for the sake of fiction, not to mention the lives of my friends, my family and complete strangers. If someone ever begins a sentence with the words 'Whatever you do, please don't breathe a word of this,' I always ask them, beg them, to go no further. *Don't tell me.* I won't be able to help myself: you'll find yourself, halfway through a dinner party or a radio interview, at the heart of an edited anecdote or worse still in a book. As the main character. I'm hopeless at keeping a secret. No need to torture me: just ask and I'll tell you. I had come to the conclusion that I was genetically programmed to tell people everything – right up until that moment.

I took a breath, considering where I should start, whether I should tell them about Max and the nipple clamps, or how after we had driven home from the restaurant – the one he'd taken me to naked – he had found a spot in the middle of nowhere and spanked me over the bonnet of his car. Or the long afternoons we had spent in my sitting room, with him tying me up, spanking me, exploring my limits. OK, so maybe not, but maybe if I mention the whole spanking thing in passing?

As it was, the words stayed wedged in my throat, unspoken. Maybe telling them about Max wasn't such a great idea after all. Maybe just keeping my mouth shut, going to Joan's do and meeting Shaun would be the easier option. We could have a quick chat over the Le Creuset display and I could give them the whole 'He's a lovely man, but not my sort of man, and maybe I'm not ready yet' speech and get off scot-free. Too late now, though.

I thought about Max and the things he had introduced me to. Was I ashamed? No. Was I afraid that they wouldn't understand? Possibly. Was I afraid that they would disapprove? Very likely – although more because of the risk than because of being narrow-minded. Would they think I was barking mad? I was almost certain of it. But what worried me most was that they might think badly of me.

All of which made no sense; I know things about them that would make your hair curl, things far juicier than any of the stuff I used in my erotic novels. They're my best and oldest friends and yes, they're judgemental, but aren't we all? I think I was afraid that if I told them they just wouldn't get it.

'He's nice,' I heard myself saying.

'Sweet Jesus,' said Gabbie, rolling her eyes. 'You really are scraping the barrel. Why don't you just admit defeat and go and meet Shaun?'

'Because I've just told you, I've met someone.'

'Who is *nice*,' chipped in Helen. 'Oh, come on, Sarah, you've got nothing to lose. You heard Joan – "lovely" trumps "nice" any day.'

I didn't want to get myself into a who-has-more-oomph argument, so I didn't say anything at all.

'Well, you know what that means, don't you?' said Helen.

'Oh no,' I groaned. 'Not yet.'

'Come on,' said Gabbie. 'You've got no one but yourself to blame – you've just outed yourself. You know the rules: once he's out he's fair game.'

We haven't got that many house rules but the ones we do have are pretty much inflexible. And one of the biggies (besides everyone bringing chocolate, cake or dessert to every get-together) is that once we've announced there is a new man in our lives we have to let the others meet him as soon as is humanly possible.

This may seem a little odd, but it's the law. It's also a real acid test. We've all made some horrible mistakes with men since becoming single, and good friends can help you save yourself the pain – if you'll listen. Good friends can help you take seriously those first impressions you tried to kid yourself were just a trick of the light. Good friends can make the judgements you're afraid to. Good friends can tell you when there's something not quite right about him. And when you take no notice of what they tell you, and it happens anyway, good friends will refrain from saying 'I told you so' until one or both of you is pissed.

'So,' said Gabbie, folding her arms across her chest in a no-nonsense way. 'What's this new man's name, then?'

'Max.'

'So far so good,' said Gabbie wryly.

'And what does he do?' asked Helen. Helen likes a man with prospects.

'It's complicated.'

'Oh my God, don't tell me: he's married,' snapped Gabbie.

'But his wife doesn't understand him,' added Helen.

'And they stopped sleeping together years ago.' Joan.

'No, no and no,' I said, holding up my hands in surrender. 'He's not married. I'm just not sure if he's anything – not really,' I bluffed, desperately trying to reel Max back in.

I should have known that that wasn't going to cut it. The ones who weren't anything aren't usually mentioned unless they are unexpectedly amazing in bed (Helen's relief postman), have some very funny habits (Gabbie's old dentist), are a dire warning (Joan's version of God) or are used as an example of how best not to be Mr Right (so that'd be all four of us, then).

Three pairs of eyes were locked on me now. I knew how it worked for potential partners, lovers and menfolk: trial by girlfriends.

'OK,' I said. 'OK, he's a business consultant, divorced, late forties, six foot something, dark hair.'

'And where does he live?'

I told them. He lived in a large village about forty minutes' drive away from my place, which was close to perfect. 'He's got his own house; he's got his oldest son living with him at the moment because he has just got back from a gap year in Australia, and he drives a Beamer.'

They all nodded in unison. It meant so far so good, but I knew them: they wanted more. A lot more.

'As well as his son he's got a grown-up daughter and another daughter by his girlfriend. They're separated. His daughter is six. I met him online. Joan was my safe call.' I nod in her direction. Joan nods her confirmation.

'I didn't realize you were going to see him again,' said Joan accusingly.

'And it's ironic, really, given that she's just tracked down Mr Right for you,' said Helen, picking at the remains of salad. 'Do you reckon that your Mr Right would do for me, Joan?'

I hoped that the spotlight had moved on but it wasn't that easy.

'How about Joan's do? You could bring Max to that,' suggested Gabbie.

'I'm not sure he's that interested in kitchen gadgets.' Unless you've got any that you can use to torment naked women, I thought.

'But he does like food?' asked Gabbie. She has this theory that men who have generous appetites for food and wine take the same generous appetites to bed with them.

I thought about eating dinner with Max – he obviously loved food – and how he laughed a lot, and I thought about how I really liked the way his eyes crinkled up when he smiled, and his generous mouth; but most of all I thought about how much he knew about women's bodies and the way his fingers and tongue made me feel, the way he made me purr and beg and gasp with pure pleasure. My impression was that he liked everything and he liked lots of it.

I realized that Gabbie was watching my face with amusement. 'So that's a yes, then, is it?' she said.

When I got home from our girls' evening in, I discovered Max had left me a message on my answering machine: 'Miss you. Hope you had a great evening. Ring me when you get in.'

Embarrassingly my heart did that funny back-flippy thing. I picked up the phone and tapped in his number. After we'd exchanged social niceties, I said, 'I don't suppose you fancy coming to a glorified Tupperware party, do you?'

He laughed. 'I'm not sure. Why, who's asking me?'

I explained about Joan's open evening, assuming that he would say no, and then added the real reason: 'My friends want to interrogate you, Sir.'

'That's to make sure that I'm not some kind of psychopath, is it?' The sound of his voice made me feel warm inside.

'Yes, Sir,' I said. Probably a bit late for that, and that's before they found out that he was a sadist.

'OK, and actually that's good, because one of the things I wanted to tell you was that we've been invited out to dinner, and I wondered if you'd like to go.'

'We have?' I said. 'By who, Sir?'

'Friends of mine,' he said.

'Right, and will they want to interrogate me?'

Max laughed. 'Highly unlikely, although they may want to tie you up.'

Which cleared up my next question.

'So shall I tell them that you'll come, Sir?' I said.

'Sure, and shall I tell my friends the same?'

I smiled. 'Why not, Sir?' I said. 'Why not?'

Chapter Eleven

'It's time to start living the life you've imagined.'
Henry James

'Do come in out of the rain, darlings. Come in, come in,' said our hostess, beckoning us inside. 'So lovely to see you again, Max, and you must be Sarah. Delighted to meet you. I've heard so much about you,' she gushed, as she embraced first Max and then me.

I wondered exactly what it was she had heard, and when I say 'hostess' I use the term loosely. Georgina was six foot four if she was an inch, built like a brick outhouse with the kind of physique most men would kill for at thirty, let alone in their early fifties. She had broad shoulders, a narrow waist and great legs, which had been waxed or shaved, as she was wearing sheer skin-tone stockings, along with the most fabulous shoes.

Georgina had huge feet, size twelve – I know because I asked her – and was wearing a pair of custom-made kitten heels. They were gorgeous, covetable, in peacock blue, and set with diamanté and little blue and turquoise stones. Her outfit was equally gorgeous: a beautifully cut cocktail frock and matching long jacket in a fabric that draped like liquid silk, matched her shoes and reached to just above the knee.

When I admired her shoes she positively purred with pleasure. 'I'm so glad you like them – I had them specially made to match my evening dress. This fabulous man makes all my shoes for me. They just have a nice little inch-and-three-quarter heel, but they still do that whole calf thing,' she said, turning her foot to the side so that I could admire her long shapely legs. 'I mean, I'd look ridiculous in stilettos,' she added, without a hint of irony. 'I have all my clothes made for me. I found this amazing little woman. Buying anything really special off the rack for a woman my size is just about impossible.'

I nodded. She seemed absolutely delighted to have another woman to talk to.

In another life, a million miles from this one, Max told me, her alter ego, Ben, was something high up in a multi-national that everyone had heard of.

'My seamstress said that just above the knee is a very flattering length for the older woman,' Georgina assured me, taking my arm and guiding me towards canapés and champagne, which were arranged on trays on a table in the centre of the huge hallway. She'd teamed the outfit with a Purdy bob in soft caramel blonde, subtle make-up and lots of jewellery, and she moved in a great cloud of Chanel No 5.

I liked Georgina the minute I clapped eyes on her. It didn't take me long to discover that she was quick, funny, candid, gossipy and a mine of information. Better still, I didn't have to wrestle with the dilemma of whether to call her Sir or Madam.

* * *

Max and I had been invited to a supper at Georgina's house with a small group of people that Max had known for years. They were into the lifestyle – that's what Max said. *The lifestyle.*

During my research online I had seen endless websites and that there is a huge industry servicing the lifestyle with sex toys, restraints, whips, canes, bondage gear, outfits, dungeon equipment, holidays, chains, and even greetings cards, gifts and soft toys. But up until Max's phone call I had assumed – wrongly, as it turned out – that as far as the whole BDSM thing went, other than the odd date *à deux* out in the vanillaverse, he and I would be keeping ourselves to ourselves. I thought that it was something that for the most part – fetish clubbers and exhibitionists aside – went on between couples in secret, behind closed doors, and that what went on between us would be happening either at my place or Max's. I hadn't really thought about going out together as a couple with my straight friends, let alone going out with any of Max's weird ones. Wrong, wrong and wrong – birds of a feather flock together. People who are into BDSM don't live apart from the rest of everyday life; rather they're part of the rich tapestry of it – it's just that they're some of the more twisted stitches.

So I had been flattered, but also really curious, when Max had asked if I wanted to go out for dinner with him, with this group of his friends who also were into BDSM.

'When you say "into", what does that mean exactly?' I asked. I had visions of me rolling up all Brad and Janet straight into a scene from *The Rocky Horror Picture Show*, complete with a dungeon full of leather-clad, whip-wielding weirdos.

'Everyone who will be there is either a Dom or a sub, and Georgina, our hostess, is a transvestite.' Which certainly chimed with the whole *Rocky Horror* thing I'd got going on in my head, although Max said it casually, in the same way you might say Georgina was a keen gardener. 'Oh, and she's gay. And a switch.'

'Which means what exactly?' I asked.

'A switch is someone who takes on the role of Dom in some situations and subbie in others. Some people would say they get the best of both worlds.'

'Have you ever wanted to switch?' I asked.

'No,' said Max. 'Although Georgina keeps telling me I shouldn't knock it till I've tried it.'

'So what do I wear, Sir?' I asked.

'It's black tie, so dress up,' he said.

'When you say "dress up", what do you mean exactly, Sir?'

'Georgina loves entertaining. Her parties are always over the top, so evening dress, heels, jewellery – knock yourself out, go to town. Something stunning would be just fine.'

'Stunning?'

'Stunning, Sir,' Max corrected. 'And no underwear,' he added, as if I needed any reminding.

I already knew that Max kept a running total of how many times I broke the rules. I suspected there was a good chance that he was writing them down somewhere.

Life had changed so much in the months since we'd met. I still couldn't walk past the side table in the sitting room without getting flashbacks of the first time we'd got together, which left me with a funny little shiver of excitement.

After our first session together I'd slipped off my dressing gown as I was about to get into the shower and had caught sight of my body in the bathroom mirror. I saw the marks across my back from the flogger, which I guessed would bruise, and the sight of them gave me an odd and unsettling sense of pride. I felt strangely peaceful after that first meeting and since I'd started to play I was sleeping the best I had for years. It was as if finding BDSM had finally joined up the random patterns of dots in my head. It felt as if I'd finally found what I was looking for.

For a couple of weeks before our dinner date at Georgina's Max had been away on business and I'd been away teaching on a residential course. Trying to talk on the phone had proved close to impossible – I'd had no mobile signal at all except in the lobby by the reception desk of the hotel where I'd been staying, which wasn't exactly the ideal place to explore the continuing mysteries of BDSM – so we'd been spending a lot of time emailing, texting and IM-ing. Writing 'Sir' is so much easier than saying it.

We spent hours online. Max liked to tease me with descriptions of what he planned to do to me. I played along and described my fantasies. Text and internet sex might not be as great as the real thing, and the fantasy element loomed large, but it was huge fun and not something I'd been expecting to be doing in my forties. And I was excited and at the same time relieved to have finally found a place to explore and try out my kinks. I was still trying to work out my feelings about pain, but if I'm honest I couldn't wait to see Max again. I had never surrendered myself so totally to anyone in my life before, and choosing to trust someone so implicitly was heady stuff. Mad? Probably. Addictive? Definitely. Dangerous? Well, yes, but nothing is without risk and in this case it was a risk I was prepared to take.

I was remarkably calm about the things Max and I had got up to. There were lots of things I didn't know about or understand, but Max assured me that it could all be learned and he would be delighted to teach me, and I wanted him to teach me.

Each time we talked on the phone, on Instant Messenger or by email I enjoyed the crackle of desire and flirtation. The connection between us was growing and I liked the way it felt. Between conversations about the niceties and otherwise of BDSM, we spent a lot of time talking about books, films, music and life in general. It sounds mad to say that it wasn't what I had expected, but it wasn't. For the first time it made me consider if I wanted a real, long-term relationship based on BDSM. Not that that was what Max was suggesting or offering, but what we had was beginning to feel like the beginning of something potentially bigger and more long-term than just a casual arrangement. I believe we both wanted more.

But whatever it was or whatever it became, Max made it perfectly clear every time we spoke, texted or emailed that we played by the rules or not at all. I wondered if it was possible to live by the rules and still have a normal relationship. What made a BDSM relationship work, he said, was keeping and respecting the dynamic of Dom and sub, Master and slave, and not coming out of role when we were together. If we didn't respect the rules, then it became not so much a game as a joke. When we were together our roles were rigidly defined. For him that was the way BDSM worked and hadn't I wanted him to guide me through the mechanics of it? But could I live like that every day? It was a thought I would return to many times.

So what do you wear to a dinner party being hosted by a six-foot-four gay transvestite and guests with assorted but unspecified kinks? I'd thumbed through my dog-eared copy of Trinny and Susannah, but they were no help at all. So I'd spent hours rifling through my wardrobe trying to work it out for myself, weighing the possibilities, trying things on. I eventually decided on the safe option: a classic little black dress that had a tight empire-line bodice and a narrow skirt – which I probably wouldn't have worn with a bra anyway – teamed with barely black stockings and suspenders, no knickers, black high-heeled strappy sandals, chandelier earrings and coral lipstick.

It was an outfit I had worn several times before and always felt good in, although up until that point always with my knickers firmly on. The lack of knickers made me very aware of my body – or more accurately feelings of nakedness and exposure, which I suspect was the whole point. The narrow skirt made me feel slightly more confident about going commando; the last thing I needed was a Marilyn moment on the way to the car.

When Max arrived he came bearing flowers and he smiled as I opened the door to him. 'You look gorgeous,' were his opening words.

I felt myself blushing as he stood back to admire me and my outfit. I also felt a little flutter of pleasure in the pit of my stomach. Fancying him was such a good feeling.

Besides the flowers – big pink peonies – he was carrying a square gift box. 'Something for you to wear,' he said, handing me the box.

I was rather hoping it contained knickers, something slinky in silk with a bit of a luxury lace thing going on – but it was soon apparent that it didn't. Instead, inside was a silver circlet made up of small, articulated plates – a necklace – with a padlock as the fastener. I picked it up and turned it over in my fingers. The whole thing was far heavier than it looked and on closer inspection the lock was quite obviously not for show, although to the untrained eye it looked like a piece of modern jewellery.

'I didn't think a studded dog collar would really go with your outfit. I'd like you to wear it all the time from now on.' He paused. 'If you're happy with the idea, that is.'

I looked up at him.

The collar was hinged at the centre point so that you could put it on, but I suspected the only way to get it off once it was locked, if you didn't have the key, was with a set of bolt croppers or to enlist someone with a talent for house breaking.

'Why don't you try it on?' he said.

I hesitated.

Max raised an eyebrow. 'Is there a problem?'

I turned the collar over a couple of times. In its own way it was beautiful. It was certainly beautifully made. On the back of the lock was engraved the words 'The property of Max –'

I'd seen collars on consensual slaves in books and BDSM sites, and I'd read about their significance. I'd been researching this world and writing about it for years, and the necklace was just a piece of jewellery, not manacles or leg irons; but what it represented was my acceptance that Max was my Dom, and if I chose to wear it I was agreeing to the notion – however preposterous – that he owned me. I reminded myself it was like the contract: it was only as binding as I believed it to be.

It was not a formal collaring – which implies permanent ownership and commitment – but it was still a symbol of possession, a commitment on both our parts to continue our journey together. I hadn't expected him to suggest it so soon, if at all.

'Is there a problem?' Max repeated.

'No, Sir.' I looked up at him. 'What does it mean?'

He smiled. 'That you and I are beginning something – and at the moment it is very new and small and fragile, and that's fine, but I wanted to mark it. I want you to wear it for me.'

I nodded, handing the collar back to him. 'It's a big thing.'

He nodded. 'As big as you want to make it. And there's no pressure. If it's too soon I can put it back in the box – no harm, no foul. There's no rush.'

'Can I wear it tonight, Sir?'

'You mean try it out?' Max said, raising his eyebrows. 'See how it feels?'

I laughed. 'Sort of, Sir.'

'OK. Here, let me put it on for you.'

The metal felt cold and heavy against my skin and I had a slight flutter as the lock clicked shut, but it also had a real erotic charge. I had agreed to the idea of submission, and this necklace was tangible proof. The expression on Max's face was a mix of delight and something altogether more proprietorial.

'It looks good,' he said. 'Here, what do you think?'

I looked into the mirror above the fireplace and reached up to touch the cool metal where it rested against my skin. The necklace looked perfect with the dress I was wearing. Standing behind me, Max ran his fingers around the front of the circlet, letting them linger on the lock, brushing my fingertips as he did. His touch sent shivers through me.

'It suits you,' he said.

I smiled. He was right: it was a subtle sign that I was something apart.

'Would you like me to take it off?' he said.

'No, Sir,' I said. 'I really like it.'

He smiled. 'I'm glad. It's time we were gone. We don't want to be late.'

'Yes, Sir,' I replied, and picking up my wrap and bag followed him out to the car.

* * *

Georgina's home – a rambling ranch-style bungalow – was tucked away behind electronic gates at the end of a long, well-manicured drive. Despite reassurances from Max that everyone was lovely and that we'd have a great evening, I was nervous – make that very nervous. He knew the people we were going to spend the evening with well, but for a newbie it was difficult to know what to expect once you got beyond the whole giant gay transvestite thing.

In the hallway Georgina handed us both a glass of champagne and beamed at me as if I was a new puppy. 'It's always so lovely to meet a fresh face. Max tells me you met on the internet. I met Anita the same way. I'll introduce you just as soon as I track her down, and you're not to worry about her: her bark is far worse than her bite. She's an absolute poppet once you get to know her. Now you are going to stay, aren't you? I'll get Barry to show you to your room. I love sleepovers – they mean that we can all relax and have a drink.'

I smiled and said nothing, while glancing across pointedly at Max.

There had to be some upside to the whole don't-speak-unless-spoken-to rule. I'd brought an overnight bag with me at Max's insistence but had already said that I would prefer to go home. Mad as it might sound, I'm a bit of a prude, and had a horrible feeling that there was a chance that Georgina's jolly dinner might degenerate into some kind of kinky swingers party. I wasn't basing that on anything Max had said or suggested, or on anything I'd seen in the few minutes since we'd arrived; it was just that I'd got no yardstick to judge these things by. Swinging was something I'd read about but had studiously managed to avoid all my adult life. I really don't mind what other people get up to, but the idea of having casual sex with complete strangers after a couple of glasses of warm Chardonnay was, and is, completely abhorrent to me. Being kinky doesn't necessarily make you broad-minded.

I didn't need to worry; Max had taken what I had said to heart. 'I'm afraid we can't tonight, Georgina,' he said, sounding genuinely apologetic. 'I've got a breakfast meeting tomorrow. Another time, though, we'd love to stay over.' News to me, but face-saving.

'Oh poop,' said Georgina, with a wave of a hand that revealed fabulously manicured bright-blue nails. 'He is such a spoilsport, isn't he? Next time I'm going to insist that you stay – is that clear?'

Max pulled a face that implied regret and then gave an almost imperceptible nod in my direction.

'Another time, then, sweetie. And I mean it. Maybe you could come over some time on your own, just the two of you. I'd planned to give you the green room. Barry and I have just given that end of the house a bit of a makeover,' Georgina was saying. Then she smiled. 'Feel free to use it while you're here, if you like, if you want to get changed or powder your nose or anything. Seems a shame not to use it – I've had Barry whip the Dyson round. Now, let me introduce you to some people, Sarah.'

I glanced round. There were around a dozen guests besides Max and me. All the men were in dinner suits, the women were dressed up to the nines in evening dresses, cocktail frocks and evening gloves, and all but one were well over forty. The exception was a tall, very slim, red-headed woman who was dressed in a dinner jacket and trousers and smoking a thin brown cigarette in a long holder.

'Ah, there you are,' said Georgina, all smiles. 'This is Anita.' The redhead moved towards us with the easy grace of a cat, and looked me up and down as though I was lunch.

Georgina raised her very nicely plucked Brooke Shields-style eyebrows. 'Play nicely, Anita. You remember Max? And this is Sarah. Sarah's new.' As if Anita needed telling.

Her gaze moving on, Anita smiled, extended a hand to Max and air-kissed him on each cheek, mwah, mwah. 'Delighted to see you again, darling. Long time no see. And this is yours, is it?' she asked, glancing in my direction. I felt a flurry of indignation but didn't say anything. Max wasn't at all fazed.

'Certainly is. Very much so,' he said, raising his glass. 'And off-limits.'

'Oh no.' Anita pulled a face. 'Really? So no sharing, then?' she asked, tipping her head to one side, flirting, feral.

He smiled wolfishly. 'Not tonight, Anita, no.'

Not tonight? What the hell did that mean? I felt my colour rising but was determined not to catch Anita's or Max's eye.

The redhead pouted. 'Oh Max, you're far too straight up and down, darling. And so greedy. Sharing makes it so much more fun, and you know how much I enjoy a little fresh meat.'

'I remember. So where exactly is Carly this evening?'

The redhead shrugged. 'What can I tell you? I've got no idea. I'm sure she must be around somewhere.'

Do I need to tell you I didn't like Anita? The things she said came straight out of a bad porn movie, and she looked sulky and like trouble.

Georgina sighed. 'Stop it, Anita. And Carly is in the kitchen.' Then, turning to us to fill in the blanks, she continued, 'She and Barry are doing the food tonight. You know Carly's a chef? She's very good. And Anita, please behave, will you?' There was a hint of rebuke in her tone.

'Oh, come on, you know you like it much better when I don't, Georgie. Anyway, I'm starving. Has everyone arrived yet? When are we going to eat?'

Georgina glanced around at the people in the room. 'I think we're just waiting for Frank and Lena now. They said they'd be here. I can't imagine they'll be very much longer. We'll give them a few more minutes and then get everyone into the dining room.' At which point something or someone caught her eye and she said, 'I'm so sorry, will you excuse me? I need to go and check on the food. Anita will make the introductions, won't you, darling?'

As soon as Georgina had gone, Anita shrugged and, ignoring us, made a beeline for the drinks table.

Max watched her walk away. I didn't say anything. I didn't need to.

'Don't mind Anita. She's mostly harmless. It's a bit of a complicated set-up here,' Max said. 'Georgina is a switch. Anita was her Dom when the two of them first got together, which I think was a couple of years ago, and Barry is her slave.'

'Anita's?'

He smiled, 'No, and that's "Anita's, Sir". No, Barry is Georgina's slave. They've been a couple for God knows how many years.'

I nodded. I'm not sure that 'complicated' was a big enough word, really. I might need a diagram. I was going to ask Max what you called a gay transvestite but it sounded like the beginning of a bad joke so didn't. 'And what about Carly, Sir?'

He smiled. 'You'll like Carly. She's another sub. I've met her two or three times now. She's lovely.'

Which wasn't quite what I meant. I wanted the dirt on what was going on and how the complications stacked up between Georgina, Anita, Barry and Carly, but then again I'm like that. Maybe I should have advertised for a gossip, not a Dom.

'So are Carly and Anita an item, Sir?'

He shook his head. 'I'm not altogether sure what's going on there at the moment. They used to be.'

Which wasn't any help at all. Max handed me another glass of champagne. 'Here,' he said. Alcohol wasn't likely to make anything any clearer.

I thanked him and settled in to people-watching. Even given the basic unorthodox set-up, so far the party was lacking in much of the way of out-and-out weirdness. Other than the fact that it was obvious that Anita was a bitch, predatory and someone who I planned to stay well clear of, and that Georgina was a man in a frock, there was nothing that untoward going on, and thanks to a glass or two of decent champagne and a couple of canapés I was quite enjoying myself. Max was relaxed and obviously at ease as he introduced me to some of the other guests.

I managed to speak only when I was spoken to, which relieved me of having to do much in the way of small talk, and gave me the time and the opportunity to watch everyone else. The other guests were charming and chatty. Yes, some of them were wearing collars and one man had a set of broad metal bracelets on, which slid out from under the cuffs of his dress shirt. And yes, some people were calling other people Sir and Madam, but it was fine, really.

We spent a disproportionate amount of time listening to a man named Kit, who cornered us over by the Pringles and had to be the world's dullest pervert. He and his wife had just bought a house that had a perfect room for a dungeon and they were waxing lyrical about a fabulous man they'd found, who supplied restraints and made big pieces of bondage equipment to order and was going to give them a quote to kit the dungeon out – although Kit planned to do some of the work himself. To be honest, this wasn't what I was expecting. I was beginning to glaze over.

There was a discussion about the straps. Leather was a no-no because Kit's wife was a vegetarian and they were looking into alternatives, because the last thing they wanted was for their dungeon to look cheap – obviously.

Kit's wife, who was Northern and very intense, was juggling a champagne flute, a side plate and a dog's lead, which was attached to the collar that Kit was wearing, and was trying to add emphasis and explanations about the dungeon work with her hands. No mean feat.

'Nylon webbing,' she said, *sotto voce*, when she caught me looking at Kit's collar and lead. 'Although he's not keen on this one. He's got a nice blue one he wears about the house but you have to wear black out, really. But this one chafes. We get them from Pets at Home; they do a really nice selection. The woman in there thinks we've got a mastiff –'

Fortunately Georgina rescued us from a discussion on the merits of eyebolts and those rubber things you strap shrubs up with by announcing that it was time for dinner.

As we followed her into the dining room, I decided that BDSM is a keen DIY-er's dream kink, and that Kit and his wife were among the top ten people I would least like to be trapped in a lift with.

The dining room was a long panelled room lit with candles in sconces. A dark wooden table ran the length of the room and was set for the whole posh dinner-party malarkey: candelabra, God knows how many glasses for different wines, jugs of water, bowls of flowers, linen napkins, and the kind of heavy ornate cutlery you usually associate with good restaurants and decent hotels.

There was also the most fabulous smell in the air. I was instantly, startlingly hungry.

The candle flames flickered in the breeze from the open door and made the cut glass glitter. It looked exquisite, luxurious and inviting, like something styled for a magazine photo shoot. There were murmurs of approval and appreciation as everyone filed in to take their seats.

Each place setting had a name card, but as my eye settled in, it looked as if someone had miscalculated, as there were far more people than chairs – which was the moment that I spotted the cushions on the floor by each place setting. Alongside some of the cushions were dog bowls.

Dog bowls? I glared at Max – no way, José. If he caught my drift or saw the look I gave him he said nothing. No one else seemed at all concerned. Fortunately – or unfortunately, given how hungry I was – there was no dog bowl by my cushion. This time Max did see my expression.

'Sit,' he said, in the same voice you'd use for the family pet.

I did as I was told, not wanting to draw attention to myself, and as I sat down I noticed that Kit was on the cushion next to mine, kneeling, resting his head against his wife's thigh while she stroked his hair and blessedly silent.

'Are you OK?' Max asked.

'Yes, Sir,' I murmured, though it wasn't exactly what I felt. In all the fantasies I'd ever cooked up over the years I'd never imagined myself sitting on a cushion on the floor at a transvestite's dinner party.

I glanced round at Georgina's other guests, both seated and curled up on their cushions.

'Don't look so worried.' He laughed. 'Relax. You're not going to be ravaged or set upon.'

I just nodded, wondering whether to ask about the food and why I hadn't got a dog bowl. To be perfectly honest, I was more interested in the food than being ravaged. I was ravenous.

It took a few moments for everyone to settle down. Georgina was seated at one end of the table, Anita at the other, still smoking. Georgina tapped her glass and did a little 'welcome to my weird soirée' speech, and then the kitchen door swung open and out came two people, carrying trays. I assumed the two people were Barry and Carly.

Barry was tiny, barely five foot two, wearing black patent Doc Martens, a pair of very shiny skin-tight PVC shorts and a spiked dog collar. He was in his mid-forties and had a great tan, multiple tattoos, a shaved head and an amazingly well-toned body that made him look as if he was entirely composed of walnuts and taut string. Alongside him was an equally diminutive blonde woman wearing the kind of hairnet you get in fast-food outlets, a matching spiked collar and nothing else – well, if you discount the nipple and labial piercings. Carly was probably in her thirties, and pretty, although to be honest I wasn't looking at her face. She had a bar and ball piercing through each nipple and her labia had a row of studs up either side: shiny stainless-steel balls like a row of ball bearings. I stared, wondering what the hell she said when she went to the doctor. Lord only knows what she would do to an airport security scanner.

The two of them moved around the table with practised ease, handing out the first course to the seated Doms, before returning to the kitchen for a tray of food that was served up into each dog bowl.

Did I feel degraded or abused at being treated like Max's pet woman? No, not at all. At any time I could have stood up and called a halt to it, but it was fun. I was happy and excited to be playing this game and enjoying the bizarre journey that Max was taking me on, trusting him to show me the sights and keep me safe. That said, I *was* getting a little bit stressed about the food. What if they weren't going to feed the people without dog bowls? And how mad was it to go to a BDSM do and worry about whether you're going to get fed or not? Worse still, some of the dog bowlers had been given the nod by their Doms and were currently tucking into their supper. I glanced up at Max.

He was busy talking to Kit's wife. She was wondering whether to go for woven hemp webbing and brass fittings in her new dungeon, for a steam punk mock-Victoriana look. I leaned my head on Max's thigh, trying to attract his attention without breaking the no-speaking rule. I wondered if yapping or whimpering would be more effective. I pressed harder. Max stroked my hair absently without actually registering what he was doing, so I whined, like a dog.

Max glanced down at me and laughed. 'What is it, Lassie? Has someone fallen down a mine shaft?'

I wish I'd bitten him.

I opened my mouth. He took a little parcel of something savoury from his plate and fed it to me. It was delicious. Tiny, but delicious. He fed me another.

This set the pattern for dinner. Hand-fed morsels from the hand of the Master. With hindsight I can see that it was meant to be erotic; the dominating partner controlling and teasing the subbie, slipping fabulous treats into their open, eager mouths, but at the time that aspect was completely lost on me because I was so hungry. I just wanted him to feed me faster and stop messing about. Meanwhile the dog bowlers were busy chomping through theirs. I think they got more. I wondered what you had to do to qualify for a bowl.

After dinner the Doms retired to the sitting room to have coffee. I could hear them from my cushion but from where I was sitting I couldn't see them.

'So this is your first time, is it?' asked Kit, finishing off a smidgeon of dessert that appeared to have been left in his bowl.

I nodded, not altogether sure what the etiquette was when it came to talking to other subbies without the Doms around and hoping that Max wouldn't be too long. The last thing I wanted was to be left alone with Kit the DIY king.

'We always have a good time here. After dinner we usually all go down to the dungeon. Barry's got a new toy he wants to show off. For suspension. I'm thinking of getting the same thing for mine. You know, in the new house. In the dungeon. Did I tell you about our plans for the dungeon?'

I groaned inwardly and wondered how much trouble I'd be in if I got up and went looking for Max.

Fortunately Max arrived before I died of boredom. 'Come on,' he said, helping me to my feet. 'Georgina is desperate for us to see the green room.'

I didn't protest.

Georgina's new guest room was at the other end of the house, and almost made me wish I'd agreed to stay. OK, so I'm a complete sucker for a nicely turned-out bedroom and a bit of luxury, and the green room did look fabulous. It was large for a bedroom, with French windows to one side overlooking a small courtyard garden. One wall had the most exquisite giant-print feature wallpaper. There was a queen-sized bed draped with a luscious, liquid, silky green canopy and a matching throw, and a great pile of matching fabulously arranged cushions and bolsters.

I know that on the whole straight men just don't get the whole cushion thing, but give me a bed piled with cushions and loads of pillows and I'm purring. Georgina had the most fabulous eye for colour and design. The only things – besides exquisite good taste – that set it apart from your average guest room were the metal rings set discreetly into the head- and footboards of the bed and into the ceiling and wall, and the number of over-large mirrors reflecting the room and the bed from every angle. Either side of the bed were side tables, and big lamps casting a mellow light on everything, which was handy as there was no hiding place from the mirrors.

At the foot of the bed was an ottoman – which Georgina informed us could be used as a toy box – covered in green Chinese printed silk and even more cushions. The wooden floor was strewn with fur rugs and there was a fireplace in one wall, flanked by campaign chairs.

It looked like the room of a gentleman traveller – if you discounted the cushions, the giant mirrors and the metal rings. The en-suite bathroom continued the green theme, and looked like a Victorian bathhouse with vintage tiles, antique fittings and piles of fluffy, thick, dark green bath sheets, along with racks of oils, bubbles and potions.

I noticed that my overnight bag and Max's leather hold-all were on one of the side tables.

'What do you think?' asked Max, as Georgina tactfully withdrew and left us to it.

'Fabulous, Sir. And the bed looks really comfy,' I said as I plonked myself down onto it. After all, Georgina had said we could use it while we were there; it would be impolite not to at least try it out. I bounced up and down a bit, ruining the whole artfully arranged cushion thing.

'You still want to go home?' Max asked. 'It's not too late to change your mind if you want, you know.'

'I've got to get back, Sir,' I said. Lovely or not, a duck-down duvet and some nice soft furnishings weren't going to be the things to quell my reservations about staying overnight with a house full of weirdos.

He nodded, as I sank back into the plush quilt.

'God, you ought to try it. This is fabulous, Sir,' I said, patting the spot alongside me.

'And not for you,' Max said, indicating that I should follow his gaze. I rolled over onto my stomach and looked over the edge of the bed. On the floor on the other side of the bed was a narrow, deep-buttoned mattress, similar to the kind of thing that comes with a futon, complete with a fur throw and a length of chain that reached from the bed frame to the floor. On the end of the chain was a dog collar. I looked up at him.

'This would be yours,' he said, in answer to my unspoken question.

There wasn't a big fluffy cushion or a silky bolster in sight. I didn't ask him if he was serious because it was obvious he was.

'Masters and subs don't sleep together. We use you and then kick you out of bed. But a good sub needs to be on hand just in case her Dom needs her in the night.'

I looked from the bed to the mattress. It was a real shame that the person most likely to be sleeping in the big comfy bed was the one least likely to appreciate the sheer theatrical beauty of it, but the idea of being used was quite a horny one. I said so, and then got up and straightened the throw and the cushions.

'Talking of being used, it's time you got changed,' Max said. 'We don't want to keep the others waiting, now do we?'

I felt a prickle of panic. Max had asked me to bring along a corset – I was already wearing black stockings and high heels – and I had done as I was told. I'd packed a leather corset that had matching knickers, but after the episode in the restaurant I wasn't sure that Max was really going to get me to wear the get-up in public.

I waited and I watched as he carefully unpacked the contents of my bag, putting the corset on the dressing table and taking a riding crop out of his holdall, and settled himself down on one of the campaign chairs to watch. I didn't move.

'We haven't got all night,' he said, waving the crop in my direction and indicating that I should undress. Self-consciously I undid my dress and peeled it down off my shoulders, using it as a shield. Mad as it may sound, I felt shy.

Max's expression softened. 'There's no need to be coy, although it is very endearing. We can stay in here all night if we really have to.'

'I'm not sure I can go out there dressed in that.' I nodded towards the corset.

He smiled. 'You will be fine, I promise, and most of the others will have changed too.'

I still wasn't sure.

'It's only hard the first time,' Max said. 'After that it will feel totally natural. Now, unless you want me to punish you, you'd better get a move on.'

'I thought you said we could stay in here all night if we have to, Sir?'

'I have to retain some semblance of being in charge. Get changed.'

I let the dress slip a little lower, my every move being closely watched. I was naked underneath except for a suspender belt and stockings. Finally I dropped the dress to the floor and instinctively crossed my arms across my chest.

Max looked me up and down appreciatively. 'Put your hands down by your sides,' he said. There was no mistaking his tone. I hesitated long enough for him to raise his eyebrows. I felt crazily exposed. His expression hardened. Slowly, I lowered my arms to my sides.

'Good girl,' he said. His voice was gentle and encouraging. 'Now turn around, nice and slowly,' he said. 'I want to look at you.'

I did as he told me, feeling my colour rising.

'Put your hands up on top of your head,' he said. 'Now turn around again. The collar suits you.'

I felt my pulse rate quicken.

'Here,' he said, eyes alight, beckoning me closer with the crop.

When I was within inches of him he put the crop across his lap and leaned forwards and kissed my navel, his hands circling my waist and pulling me closer still. One finger slid between the lips of my sex, seeking a way in. I gasped as my body opened up for him. He pulled away, slipped the finger into his mouth and sucked it. 'You taste divine,' he said, and then he stood up. He was still dressed in his dinner suit while I was in nothing but stockings, suspenders and high heels.

The contrast was striking. He stroked my face and cupped my breasts, caressing my nipples. I felt my stomach flutter.

'You're gorgeous,' he murmured. 'Absolutely stunning.'

Max made me feel beautiful, and the undisguised look of pleasure on his face confirmed it. Desire and sexual confidence are not about perfection or being a size eight, they're in your head. My head was full.

He picked up my corset from the dresser. It was made from butter-soft black leather, strapless, boned, with hooks and eyes all the way down the front and laces at the back to tighten it up with. Max unfastened my suspender belt, took it off and rolled my stockings down to my knees, before wrapping the corset around me and fastening the hooks one by one, taking his time, stroking me as he did, fingers and lips pressed to every inch of me – my belly, the rise of my ribs, the soft skin between my breasts, my collarbones, my neck. There was no part of me that escaped his caress.

I felt like a toy, being dressed and caressed, turned this way and that. Getting dressed had never felt so sexy. My body was responding to his every touch. When the corset was fastened, Max bent down to attach the stockings to the suspenders on the corset, his fingertips trailing up the inside of my thigh. I shivered as he stroked between my legs, with feathery caresses. Before I could respond, he turned me around to tighten the laces.

A boned corset gives you great posture and an hourglass figure with very little effort, as long as you don't want to breathe. Max pulled the laces through the holes, getting them even, and then pulled them tighter, making me gasp.

'Breathe in,' he said.

I did and he pulled the cords tighter still. 'Relax. Don't fight it. Just breathe in gently and I'll take up the slack.'

I tried. The laces tightened a fraction more. In the mirror I could see my reflection. The corset emphasized every curve.

'More,' he said.

I did as he asked. 'Easy for you to say, Sir,' I gasped.

Max let the laces slacken a fraction. 'Bend over the side of the bed. Hands flat on the mattress.'

I stared at him.

'Now,' he snapped. There was, I noticed, always a change of pace when we were playing, like a gear change, when we would move from something soft and easy to something richer and deeper and more sexually charged. While the dynamic never changed, the intensity did.

As I did as I was told, I heard him opening the holdall and guessed what was coming. I had seen the riding crop earlier, laid casually across his lap, but I hadn't seen the flogger and for some reason I assumed that that was what he was getting out. Hadn't he said it was his favourite? I shivered as I heard something swish through the still air and braced myself, waiting for the kiss of the suede fronds.

The sensation was nothing like what I had anticipated, nothing at all. It was tight and fierce, like a hot bee sting that cut into my flesh, and it made me shriek and swing round to see what it was.

'Stand still,' Max said sharply, and remarkably I did. 'I want you to count the strokes.'

'It hurts, Sir,' I gasped.

'Count the strokes,' he repeated. 'Have you been caned before?'

'No, Sir,' I hissed. Caning – that certainly explained the pain.

'Ten strokes. Count for me.'

'One,' I said, hastily, wondering if I'd be able to stand it. I was already turned on. I wanted him desperately and wanted the next part of the game, but this was so raw – so cruel that it took my breath away.

He hit me again.

'Two,' I shrieked. This pain was altogether more fearsome and less bearable than either the flogging or spanking. I heard the cane cutting through the air and tensed before it hit home – which probably made it worse. The third stroke was as painful as the first and slightly harder. I knew Max would measure the strokes, building up the intensity, encouraging me to tolerate more pain with each strike, but this felt like too much right from the start.

'Don't move,' he said again, most insistently this time. 'It's important that you stay very still.'

I tried my best, but the fourth brought tears to my eyes. By the fifth stroke I was screaming, 'Lead, lead, lead, I hate this, it hurts, it hurts.' The tears were running down my face. And Max stopped. Just like that, and catching hold of me he held me tightly against his chest.

'I know, I know,' he said, in a soothing voice.

'How can you know?' I snorted. 'Why do I want to do this? It's mad.' Unexpectedly I started to sob. It felt as if I had failed, which was crazy, crazy, crazy. 'I'm so sorry,' I spluttered. 'I'm sorry.' *What was I sorry about?*

'It's all right,' he said, kissing my hair and stroking it off my face. 'We're exploring this together. It's fine to say that you want to stop. That's the whole point of having the safe words. I want you to enjoy this but I need to find out the edges of this, to find out how far we can go.'

'I'm sorry,' I heard myself saying again. *Sorry for what, for fuck's sake?*

He held me. 'Don't be sorry. You've nothing to be sorry for.'

I knew that.

I felt his excitement. I knew how turned on he was by controlling me, by tying me up, by beating me, by seeing me in pain and in pleasure. The torturer's gift is both to give pain and having the power to withdraw it, so he became both tormentor and rescuer. It was a heady combination.

The pain in my buttocks was still there, hot and angry as a burn. I looked up at him. 'It really hurt.'

Max nodded, his expression impassive.

'I think it was the shock as much as the pain. Five is nothing, is it?' I said, wiping the tears off my face. 'I wimped out, but it hurt. I hated it. I really, really hated it.'

I took a minute. I ran my fingers through my hair, trying to regain some sense of composure and control. I could see myself in the mirror: I was undone, unravelled by the pain. Then Max put his hand under my chin and tipped my face up towards him.

'Five more,' he said, his gaze holding mine.

Five more strokes, to play out some weird act of trust, some great act of submission, to give Max the power over me, to give the power back to him. I took a breath. Five more seemed like a mountain to climb. He waited.

This was a big ask; Max was asking me to push myself beyond what I thought I was capable of. I could easily have said no, but part of me understood that this was about giving myself over to him, trusting that he knew what I really could cope with, training me to go further. In many ways it was a test of how much I trusted him with the submissive part of my nature.

'Five more,' I repeated.

He nodded.

Stepping out of his arms, I stood up and took my place back over the bed. He gave me a moment or two to still myself. I willed myself to relax, trying to slow my breathing, trying to send myself into the still calm sea that had swallowed me before when he had beaten me with the flogger.

'Go with it,' Max said softly.

Easy to say, hard to do. I tried not to tense as I heard him take a practice swing, and then he hit me again.

'Six,' I gasped. The pain was no less, but this time I knew I was in control. I could have called a halt; I could have said enough was enough and Max would have stopped. But I didn't. Instead, I stepped into pain. I heard someone say seven; it must have been me. Eight, nine – I was in free fall now, the pain like a white light. The safe words hung in my mind, bright as stars, within easy reach, but I didn't say them; instead, gasping, crying out, I let myself fall into the sensations, gasping and struggling before finally drowning in them. This time surrender was easier.

Ten, and I am home and it is over.

In the stillness that followed Max dropped the cane onto the bed alongside me. I could feel my legs trembling as I waited for him to set me free. Moments passed.

'You are so beautiful,' he murmured. My posture softened.

'And you've got the cutest little row of cat's whiskers across your arse,' he whispered, his voice thick with excitement and amusement as he stroked me with his fingertips. His touch was as cool and welcome as iced water. I could hear how turned on he was.

I turned to glance over my shoulder and caught sight of my bum in the dressing-table mirror and the raised row of welts across my backside – maybe not quite cat's whiskers, but close – and understood now why Max wanted me to stand still. They would bruise: there was no doubt about that. I tipped my bum up to get a better view.

Max stepped up close behind me, and grabbing hold of my hips pulled me back towards him. My backside was glowing red hot, adrenaline coursing through me. My whole body was trembling and I was aching for release. Instinctively I thrust back into him, tipping my pelvis. I wanted him and I knew damn well that he wanted me. He pulled back a little and ran his hand over the welt marks.

I knew that with those stripes across the pale white skin of my backside, nothing short of getting dressed again was going to hide what we had been up to.

But for the moment my attention was on persuading Max to stop stroking the cane marks and to fuck me. I brushed myself against his groin and started to flex my hips backwards and forwards.

I heard him laugh. 'You are a bad, bad girl, Sarah,' he said, 'You know the rules. We agreed, remember? No sex.'

'Oh, fuck the rules,' I growled. 'And anyway that was me, it was me who said no sex.'

'And I agreed,' he said.

'Please, Sir –'

'No,' he said, sliding his hand between my legs. I was so wet and so excited that the lightest touch made me gasp. How could he say no to so willing a partner? His fingertips stroked the hard, throbbing bud of my clitoris, sending wave after wave of pleasure rolling through me.

'Don't you want to, Sir?' I gasped. Everything I'd seen in his eyes and heard in his voice suggested that he was as turned on as I was.

'It's not about what I want. It's about what we agreed.'

He turned me by the shoulders and rolled me over onto the bed. I was horny as hell, struggling to breathe from the constriction of the corset and the endorphin rush, and desperate for him. 'Please,' I murmured.

I felt his eyes moving over my body, drinking me in. 'We don't negotiate a change that fundamental while we're playing. Do you understand?'

Of course I understood. I was turned on, not deaf. Max stood between my legs; his eyes were dark with desire, a smile playing on his lips. I didn't need any more confirmation that he wanted me as much as I wanted him; everything about his body language, his face and expression echoed and amplified my desire. The difference was that he had the power to deny himself and me. And he had denied me for so long. His self-control was astonishing, and totally and completely infuriating.

'You understand, Sarah?'

'Yes, Sir.'

He took my hand and helped me to my feet. We stood in front of the mirror that was above the dressing table.

'Look at you,' he whispered. 'Just look.'

I barely recognized the person I saw in the mirror, wild-eyed, glowing skin, crazy bed-head hair and a look of wanton hunger that I had never known I possessed.

'Here,' he said, taking my hand. 'I want you to touch yourself. Show me how you like to be touched.'

I hesitated, resisting sharing something so very intimate and so very personal with him. I could feel my colour rising, but this time he wasn't taking no for an answer. His hand guided mine down over my belly, down to the swell of my sex, and pressed my fingers down onto the swollen bud of my clitoris.

I closed my eyes, feeling the sensations radiating out. His fingers pressed harder. 'Open your eyes,' he said. 'I want you to watch yourself doing this. I want to see your eyes.'

I blushed, heat rushing through me as his fingers worked with mine, caressing, circling, opening me up, exploring, stoking the fire that had already been lit. As I began to move against him, he bit my neck, cupped my breasts, nipping and tugging at my nipples while one hand shadowed mine, stroking and teasing.

I was stunned by what I saw reflected: the way my body moved against his, my face and the look in my eyes. I leaned back against Max, his fingers and mine working in tandem.

I am engulfed in his arms, safe and gasping for breath as the waves of pleasure build and roll through me. I am a breath away from orgasm when his fingers take over, an echo of mine, and I am lost, and as I look into the mirror and see what he sees in my face.

I lean against him as the pleasure rolls on and on until I beg him to stop, the sensations too much, and finally I close my eyes, breathing hard and totally, totally sated. I can feel Max's arms still around me. I can sense the heat of his body and the subtle scent of his aftershave mixed with the raw scent of his body.

How can he resist taking this to the next level? Why doesn't he want to fuck me? I'm as tormented as I am frustrated. My mouth waters. He smells wonderful. I want him to feel what I have felt, to share the sense of release, to feel him inside me, so I turn around and rest my head against his shoulder, slipping my arms around his waist.

'Please,' I murmur. 'Don't you want to?'

I can feel the taut strength of his body, the muscles in his back – but not for long.

'You know the rules, Sarah. You helped write them,' he says, gently but firmly disentangling himself. 'Come on, it's time to go. Georgina will be wondering where we've got to.' He smiles. 'You can wear your knickers if you want to.'

The man is all heart.

Chapter Twelve

'Sex is dirty only when it's done right.'
Woody Allen

Barry is a great fan of tight bondage. That's what Georgina told me as we all made our way down to the dungeon, which rather disconcertingly she referred to as the playroom.

Bondage *and* suspension, she said, which she assured me was very good for Barry's back. 'You should try it some time. It's absolutely fabulous, really. My chiropractor swears by it. We had him round to try it out over Christmas. Get Max to bring you over. You're welcome any time,' she said cheerily.

Barry was planning a demonstration for their guests.

'And then he just likes to be left there. Sometimes I leave him tied up all night – not suspended, obviously. He loves it.' Georgina paused and sighed. 'It can get a bit boring, to be perfectly honest; he's no company when he's like that and I've told him he can't use the sleep sack when he's sleeping with me. Black leather. We bought it in the States. It zips right up, over his face and everything.' She mimes. 'It's like waking up next to a chrysalis.'

Georgina's dungeon was in a large room behind the kitchen, which I guessed was probably once a double garage. There was a small separate chill-out area with comfy chairs and a sofa, a little bar, and behind that a couple of showers and a changing room. Georgina pointed out that it had a separate entrance to the rest of the house and a double bedroom in the roof space.

Just inside the door of the playroom was a long shelf on which stood bowls and baskets containing condoms, sachets of lube, rubber gloves, sanitizing spray, little sealed packets with dental dams inside, sterile swabs and a disposal box for sharps. There was a cartoon poster explaining the virtues of safe sex alongside a first-aid kit and a water cooler.

Georgina explained that she and Barry rented it out to friends; apparently lots of people rented it just for an afternoon or evening or occasionally weekends. BDSM couples aren't necessarily in traditional relationships with each other and need a safe and discreet place to play, although, she said, at the moment they were only hiring it out to friends and people who came from personal recommendations. Georgina told me that the playroom was their pension plan. I wasn't sure if she was joking, or if she was telling me all this because I'm a writer or because I was new or because she was hoping that Max and I were prospective customers. She said that she'd give me the address of their website before we left and asked if I wanted to join their mailing list. I didn't.

In the hiatus between coffee and our trip to the green room, almost all the guests had changed and the vast majority had shed a lot of their clothes. Only Georgina and Max were still dressed in the outfits they'd begun the evening in – Georgina in her cocktail frock, Max in black tie.

Kit, the DIY king, was now wearing lederhosen with braces, boxing boots and a dog collar. He looked as if he had been recently waxed and spray tanned. Mrs Kit still had him on a leash. She was tiny and wearing a scarlet corset, seamed stockings, a leather cap, gauntlets and thigh boots. Some of the other women were in corsets; one Dominatrix was in a long slinky evening dress and fur stole that wouldn't have looked out of place on Cruella de Vil. The male Doms' dress was more varied. One had leather chaps on over a posing pouch and a fringed waistcoat. One man was dressed in riding breeches and a white peasant-style shirt with an open frilly front and gathered sleeves. One was in what looked like a strong-man costume, bare-chested and in tight three-quarter trousers with braces. Here, I realized, you could be anything that you wanted to be. Glancing across at Max I wondered what his fantasy get-up looked like, or maybe black tie *was* his thing, a sort of James Bond with a whip vibe. As soon as he gave me permission to speak again I planned to ask him.

At first glance the playroom, which was painted Chinese red and had thick grey carpet tiles, big mirrors and subdued lighting, looked a lot like an upmarket gym. There were areas with large padded wipe-clean crash mats on the floor and the walls, wall bars, things hanging from the ceiling and bits of freestanding equipment that looked a lot like resistance machines – until you noticed the cuffs, ropes, chains and leg irons.

Barry was busy being tied up by Carly on one of the crash mats. He had a ball gag slung loose around his neck, which Carly explained she would put in place and tighten once she was sure Barry was happy. He needed to be comfortable, she said. 'Comfortable' was not a word I would have used. His arms were held together in a long single leather cuff – like a triangular tube – that extended from wrist to elbow and his legs were tied from thigh to ankle in a complex pattern of knotted rope. Carly was practising Japanese rope bondage, Georgina told me in a stage whisper. They had sent off for a DVD that had a step-by-step guide on it, and they'd been working their way through it.

Alongside Barry, the rope and the cuffs were the mechanics of suspension.

Meanwhile the other guests were happily making use of the various bits of equipment around the playroom. It crossed my mind that tonight might be a sales drive to promote Georgina's dungeon. There were some fliers in a basket by the water cooler and contact details for a kink-sympathetic carpenter were Blu-Tacked to the wall just inside the door. In one corner a plump blonde in a fabulous gold and black corset was settling herself into a set of stocks, assisted by her partner, who was wearing black leather trousers and a black rollneck. He looked like the man who used to abseil into a lady's bedroom to deliver a box of Milk Tray.

'Not too tight, darling?' Leather Trousers asked, as he lowered the top half of the stocks into place. The neck and wrist holes were padded and covered in dark red leather. The woman turned her head and smiled up at him. 'Lovely,' she said.

On the other side of the room one of the men was being handcuffed face down over what looked a bit like a wooden vaulting horse. His female Dom strapped his ankles to either side of the box and got a driving whip out from a selection of implements lining one of the walls. To be honest, I didn't know where to look next.

On the crash mat Carly was busy finishing off a series of very neat, regularly spaced knots. 'Barry does a lot of yoga,' confided Georgina, as Carly popped the ball gag into his mouth and tightened the strap. 'I find it a bit of a job getting down there these days. We're thinking about having a nice table made, now that we've got the electric hoist – much safer and more reliable than the old block and tackle. And Carly is an absolute treasure. We're so lucky to have found her.'

Georgina made her sound like a benign cleaning lady.

The playroom was a long, long way from sitting at home at my desk writing about BDSM. What struck me as I watched was that once you got past the leather and straps Georgina's guests weren't strange. They were a mix of ordinary people, the same people that you might see at any party. They looked like everyone else, certainly not monsters or freaks, and not at all inhibited or self-conscious about their dress or lack of it.

It was oddly refreshing and not in the least bit sordid, which before meeting them I was worried it might be. They were consenting adults who had found a safe place and like

minds to explore their fantasies with and were hurting no
one, and now, against all the odds, I was one of them.

I'd come an awfully long way since meeting Max. I
smiled to myself – Joan's do at the barns was going to be
an interesting contrast.

Max, Georgina and I watched as Barry was very slowly
lifted up on an electronic hoist. He was suspended hori-
zontally, face down, from a selection of long bars, straps
and rings. Other guests glanced our way but – for the
most part – were already absorbed in their own games.
Watching, I soon discovered that other people don't play
with other people unless invited; one of the guests was
watching while another man strapped his wife into a
standing frame with arm and leg restraints, and after a
while was invited to touch and then flog her.

It was all terribly polite and initially at least quite
tentative; strange too that the second man talked almost
exclusively to the other Dom, not the submissive woman
he was busy walloping – the eye contact and conversation
excluded the sub – and this certainly wasn't about gender,
because the chap over the horse was silent and had his eyes
downcast while his partner chatted away to another Dom
about a place she'd discovered online for American imports
of various must-have dildos. No one was having sex.

I asked Georgina about it as Barry made slow, stately
progress up towards the ceiling. Barry's expression was
blissful, as if he was on the edge of sleep.

Swapping partners and having full sex with someone
other than the person you brought with you was extremely
unusual, said Georgina, or at least that was her experience

of these kind of mixed parties (by mixed she meant hetero- and homosexual), though the edges were not as clearly defined as you might imagine, and occasionally an extra man or woman was invited to make up a threesome, but not often in these kind of open public parties. People did touch other people and there was often oral sex between consenting non-couples, she said, all very matter of fact, and she was sure that swapping did go on, but not at public parties.

'And not here. We're fine with whatever people want to do – live and let live. But we're not really into orgies,' she sniffed, apparently slightly affronted. 'At least not these days' – and then, grinning, she added that gay parties were a lot wilder.

Max listened with an amused expression as I interrogated Georgina, but didn't interrupt or reprimand me for talking without permission. I was curious to know why Georgina and Barry were so actively involved with straight couples, as I'd rather assumed that, being gay, they would stick to gay BDSM. Georgina didn't seem to have an answer and as we were speaking took a riding crop from a selection in an umbrella stand and flexed it thoughtfully. By this stage Barry was up around waist height. The hoist was quite slow, the movement smooth and even.

'Barry likes a bit of bastinado,' Georgina said conversationally in answer to what I can only assume was me raising my eyebrows. I had absolutely no idea what bastinado meant.

Carly stepped away and took hold of the frame up by Barry's head, and Georgina stepped up to the mat. She trailed the folded leather end of the crop across Barry's muscular back. He shivered and closed his eyes in what looked like ecstasy. I saw him settling, drinking in the sensations. I guess he knew what was coming next. Georgina stroked him with the crop again, and this time she trailed it down along his side, up across his calf. I realized that I was holding my breath.

I caught Max's eye. He reached out and touched my cheek, eyes bright. 'I know this is a lot to take in,' he said in an undertone. 'But you're doing really well and nothing is going to happen that you don't want to. Really. You're safe. I promise.'

I believed him.

On the mat, Georgina swished the crop back and forth a few times as if gauging the swing. It cut through the air, and then she cracked it across the soles of Barry's feet. The strength of the blow shocked me. I might have shrieked, I'm not sure, but I do know that Barry gasped with pain and I gasped with him.

Barry grimaced, his eyes widening and then snapping tight shut. The sound of the leather crackling across his feet momentarily stopped all the other players in their tracks, and they turned to look at him. No one seemed at all surprised or shocked, and an instant later they carried on doing what they were doing. I tried to imagine how it must feel. My own backside was still sore from the caning. No one had mentioned the cat's whiskers, which despite my knickers I knew were painfully obvious, but then I saw that several of the other subs had bruises and welts of their own.

As if sensing my shock, Max rested a hand in the small of my back. His touch was comforting. I tried to remind myself that this was something that Barry enjoyed, even though it was hard to believe. I'm certain that I would have passed out if anyone had hit me that hard.

Carly held on to the suspension frame so that it didn't move too much as Georgina flicked the crop back and hit Barry again. Barry let out a long, ragged, ramshackle breath. This time no one looked round.

The crop struck again and Barry's eyes snapped open. They were glazed and glassy now. I recognized the expression on his face – I'd seen it on my own. He was slipping down into the pain. Under my breath I counted each stroke – eight in all – and then Georgina was done and waved Carly over to get Barry down and untie him. She was worried that he looked uncomfortable. I didn't know how she could tell.

I asked Max. Rules or no rules, I couldn't help myself.

'She's watching him; she knows him,' he whispered. 'A good Dom watches his subbie all the time to see how they are coping. The more you play, the more you understand and the more in tune you get with each other. Georgina can read him. Now, do you want to play too or do you just want to watch?' he asked.

I felt a rush of panic. I'd barely got used to the idea of playing in private, let alone in front of strangers. It must have shown on my face, because Max shook his head and smiled. 'It's OK. Just relax. There's no pressure. I know that all this is new to you. We can take all the time you need. My plan was to fasten you to the wall and let you watch tonight, but I wanted to give you the chance to play if you wanted to. But there is no rush and no one here would dream of touching you without my permission. Do you understand?'

I nodded, and then corrected myself. 'Yes, Sir.'

'Good girl. Come with me.'

Along the back wall there were heavy metal rings set into the brickwork at various heights. Max took a set of cuffs from a selection fastened along a rope and started to unbuckle them as I watched nervously.

On the wall on a shelf above the baskets of condoms were a selection of dildos and strap-on cocks that varied in size from oh-yes via good-lord to bloody-hell and then alongside them were other things that defy description or identification. Georgina caught me looking at them and smiled.

'You can try anything you want, dear,' she said with a wave of the hand. 'Just help yourselves.'

At which point I said the first thing that came into my head, which was, 'They must be hell to keep clean.'

'Not at all, sweetie,' said Georgina, helping herself to a cup of water from the cooler. 'Barry just pops them all in the dishwasher.'

Max fastened me to the wall. 'You'll be perfectly safe,' he assured me as he buckled the straps tightly around my wrist.

He leaned in closer and kissed me on the forehead. 'Don't look so worried. I'll be here all the time,' he said, nodding towards a frame made up of crossed timbers set with wrist and leg restraints. 'Anita's gone off somewhere. She's asked me if I want to play with Carly.' He paused. 'I want you to watch.'

I stared at him in stunned silence, astonished to realize that what I felt was not relief but jealousy.

'OK?' he asked.

'Are you serious?' I whispered, oblivious to breaking the Sir rule.

'Absolutely.'

'Have you played with Carly before?'

Poker face, he nodded. 'Once or twice.'

'Was she – is she – your subbie as well?' I asked. My voice had an unexpected crackle of emotion in it, which surprised me. I was supposed to be a grown-up, but I felt exposed and cheated. I thought Max and I would only be playing with each other. For me these were all new things, and they were big things, not a trivial game, and here we were, and Max was off planning to do them with someone else. We're not a couple in a traditional sense, I reminded myself, and he won't be having sex with her. It shouldn't matter. It really shouldn't, but it does. It really, truly does.

I blinked back a flurry of unexpected tears, making an effort to pull myself together. Damn, damn, damn. I knew fancying him would mess things up.

'Would you rather I blindfolded you?' he asked, and if I saw a hint of mischief in his expression I didn't register it.

I glared at him. 'No, I bloody well wouldn't,' I snapped.

Max raised his eyebrows; it was the wrong thing to say. He pulled a blindfold from his jacket pocket. I groaned.

He smiled. The amusement in his eyes was the last thing I saw before the lights went out.

I had no idea what Max did to Carly; I certainly heard her gasp; I heard the crack of the crop and strained to pick out the sound of his voice. My best guess is that he did nothing at all, because that was the kind of man Max was. It was a test, and I had failed, or passed, and he was a sadist. I have no idea how long he left me there. It felt like for ever, while I listened to the most bizarre radio play ever written. When he took the blindfold off, Carly was still tied to the frame. Anita was beating her with a riding crop. Max was smiling.

Did Max enjoy seeing my reaction to him saying that he was going to play with Carly? I'm sure he did. Doms feed on a sense of power and control. Did he do it to be spiteful or manipulative? No, even as a sadist Max really wasn't wired that way. He did it because he could; while I trusted him implicitly he liked to wrong-foot me on occasions – but never with the important things. What it did make me realize was just how much I cared about him. I wanted him for myself, and that did come as a shock.

Chapter Thirteen

'When I have so corrupted this fragile thing and
brought out a writhing, mewling, bucking,
wanton whore for my enjoyment and pleasure, at
that moment she is never more beautiful to me.'

Marquis de Sade

'Have you had lots of Dom/sub relationships, Sir?' I asked
Max on the long drive home. It was late and I was tired and
worried that I sounded like a whiny teenager asking how
many girlfriends a new boyfriend has already had, and how
much they meant to him. I've always been convinced that
women are their own worst enemies in relationships: we
want to know everything about the man we're dating and
then torture ourselves with what we find out.

The awareness that I wanted a committed relationship
with Max was just sinking in. The thing with Anita and
Carly had really hammered it home, and I wondered where
that left me. What if he didn't feel the same way, and, if he
did, how would I integrate BDSM into my real everyday life?

Max had declared an amnesty so that we could discuss
the evening without me getting into trouble for talking,
but not on the Sir thing: the Sir thing stayed. If I miss any
out as I'm typing 'Sir', trust me: they were all there, every

last one. Max was right: it was beginning to become second nature.

Max nodded thoughtfully. 'Since my divorce, all my relationships have had a D/s element to them.'

It was raining hard; he was concentrating on the road. In the light from oncoming headlights I was struck by how strong his features were, his cheekbones, the laughter lines around his eyes; he looked good in a DJ, the formality of it suited him, and I got a sense of what he must have looked like when he was young, when he was with Eva, and there was a part of me that wished I had known him then.

'Were all of them submissives? Or did you go around converting nice girls, Sir?' I joked.

I watched his face as he considered his answer. 'It took me a while to work out exactly what submissive meant,' he said after a moment or two. 'And you have to remember that Eva found me. I wasn't sure that I would ever find anyone else like her. She changed the way I looked at everything.' He paused. 'I know you've read a lot and written a lot about the lifestyle, Sarah, so it's hard for me to gauge what you know and what you really understand about it. You know what vanilla is?'

I nodded. 'An ordinary straight relationship, with no kinks, Sir? Missionary position, lights out ...'

'OK, well, vanilla doesn't do it for me.'

'Not at all, Sir?'

'No, not at all. After Eva I made the mistake of thinking I could just go back there, go home, but I can't. It's something that you need to understand.'

'And you're happy with that?'

'Yes, and that's "happy with that, Sir".'

OK, so maybe I forgot one. I stared at him, imagining all the things that a relationship entailed: cuddling and snuggling up together on a Sunday morning reading the papers, listening to *The Archers*, gardening, having friends round for lunch, cooking and holding hands, walking the dog or sitting on the sofa, arms round each other, watching a weepie. Surely Max couldn't mean *all* those things?

'But I like vanilla, Sir,' I said.

'I know you do.' He paused. 'I asked her to marry me.'

'Who? Eva?'

Max nodded. 'I was young. I thought it would work. She'd spent a lot of time training me to be the Dom she needed, showing me what she liked; I thought it was what she wanted. She was the one who showed me what women enjoy, how to touch them, how to beat them, how to read them.'

I stared at Max's face, picked out in silhouette.

Not all women, I thought; only the ones who liked what she liked – the submissive ones. I should be grateful to Eva for everything she had taught Max and everything that they had shared, but all I could think was that somewhere deep down Max had never really got over her.

'Once I understood, I used to go to the club with Eva every chance I could,' Max said. 'She worked behind the bar there when they needed her, and when she was certain that I wouldn't bottle out she got me on the stage – masked, flogging her.' He grinned. 'She was such an exhibitionist. If anyone had ever found out in the office,

I'd have been in deep shit. Anyway, we played a lot, we went to some parties, other clubs. We met other people who were into the same thing. But she was right about me. She recognized what I was.'

'And you loved her?'

'Totally. You know what it's like at that age: everything is all consuming. Looking back now, I'm not sure now whether it was love or obsession, but whatever it was it was powerful stuff. One night I did the whole thing, bought her red roses, cooked dinner, bottle of wine, the whole shebang, and she walked in and took one look at me and said, "Whatever you're planning, Max, don't do it." Then she told me in no uncertain terms that she had no plans to be anyone's wife. She said it would be like caging a tiger.

'But instead of just carrying on as we were – which she would have been happy to do – I was angry with her. I suppose I felt rejected. I wanted more. I wanted all of her, and all of her wasn't on offer. She said that you couldn't live the lifestyle all day and every day, as you'd be exhausted and it would end up being ordinary, and she didn't want what we had to be ordinary.

'So I came home for a few days. I had intended to come home and tell Nola it was over and tell everyone about Eva, but when I got back home Nola was waiting for me. And she issued me with an ultimatum: either we got engaged or she was going to call it a day. She was tired of waiting.' Max shook his head.

'Looking back, I was a complete moron. I should have said, "Fine, go," but at the time I was young and stupid and missing Eva, and I suppose I wanted to punish Eva for saying no.'

'So you married Nola?'

He nodded. 'Something I'm not exactly proud of. She was a really good person and she certainly deserved a lot better than me. My mother really loved her. And she was a good wife and a great mother.'

'And vanilla?'

'To the core. But I thought that I could handle it, and that if I didn't feed it then the side of my nature that Eva had shown me would just fade, so Nola and I settled down and had the kids.'

'And lived happily ever after?'

Max laughed. 'Evidently not. But that wasn't her fault: it was mine. It was always there and she knew it. She said being away had changed me and she was right. When the next overseas contract came up she wanted to stay at home to be close to her family. I tried to explain to her that that was where the money was and that she could come with me – but I knew after the first time she hated it.'

'So how long were you married?'

'Fifteen years. After that first overseas contract I got after we were married, her mum and dad helped us to buy a house in the same village as them. And before you ask, yes, I was faithful all the time we were married, totally and utterly faithful. But whatever it was that Eva had seen was always there. I tried to play with Nola, but she just thought it was stupid. Then one day I came back from a contract in Dubai and Nola told me she wanted out. I hadn't seen it coming. I thought I'd been holding it together, but she said we should never have got married and that I was never really there. When I thought about it afterwards, I knew she was right. And after the shock and the practicalities of splitting up, the main feeling I had was one of relief. As soon as it was all sorted out, I went back to the town where I'd had my first overseas job.'

'To find Eva?'

Max shook his head. 'No, not to find Eva – or at least not just to find Eva. I had the chance to go back and work there and I took it. The first night I arrived I went to the club.' He shook his head ruefully and laughed. 'It was a restaurant. I went to some of the other bars we used to hang out in, but so many things had changed. There were lots of clubs, and it all looked wilder and crazier than it had back then, but there were far more posers than players.'

'And did you find her?'

He nodded. 'It took me a while, but yes. I met Jessa first: she was running one of the bars, and she told me that Eva was married and that she had an address. So I went to find her.'

'She was married?'

'Yes, but I wanted to see her. I wasn't trying to tempt her away or anything like that. Anyway, I rang and said I was back and asked if we could meet up. She was really pleased to hear from me. She was a real housewife, out in the suburbs. Really happy. I was surprised, but I was also glad.' He laughed. 'She looked amazing and glowing, and she also had a very selective memory. When we talked about the good old days she seemed to have forgotten most of it. She wasn't into anything, not living the life; her husband didn't even know. He was in IT. They had two kids and she talked about the whole thing as if it was someone else.' Max sounded sad.

'So she could do vanilla?'

'Seems so.' Max was quiet.

I wasn't sure whether to speak and if so what to say. I was thinking about vanilla relationships and what they meant to me.

'But you're warm and funny and great company,' I began, and then I stopped, not altogether sure where I planned to go with this. 'Don't you miss having real relationships?'

Max laughed. 'I do have real relationships. They're just different from the ones you're used to.'

It was late when we finally got back to my house. Max opened the car door for me and walked me up to the front door. As we got to the porch there was a moment when we both hesitated; it felt as if we were waiting for something.

'Goodnight,' Max said after a moment or two, tipping my chin up so that I was looking into his eyes. His touch sent a shower of sparks through me. 'Thank you for coming with me tonight. Georgina is one of my oldest friends.'

'Thank you for inviting me, Sir. It was interesting.'

'Interesting? Yes, I suppose it was,' he said. 'I'm glad you found it interesting.'

There was a moment of stillness and I felt the crackle of desire in the air between us.

'I'll call you tomorrow,' Max said, turning to leave. 'We can arrange for me to be interrogated by your friends.'

'You could come in if you want to,' I said, pushing open the door. 'Have coffee?' I hesitated. 'Stay,' I added.

Max shook his head.

'I could always sleep on the floor.'

Max smiled. 'Sweet dreams, Sarah,' he said, and kissed me on the top of the head before walking back to his car.

I watched him pull away and then headed into the house, surprised at how very empty and quiet it felt without him.

Chapter Fourteen

'Your body is the church where Nature asks to be
reverenced.'
Marquis de Sade

The shop where Joan works is in a very handsome old barn
complex, which is owned by two brothers. Surrounded by
mature trees and lush landscaping, there's a fabulous café,
great food in the deli, a craft shop, a guy who makes
leather handbags, another who makes silver jewellery, and
then in the main barn all these lovely kitchen things, all
brilliantly styled and lit – with price tags to match. Two
or three times a year the brothers hold promotional
evenings with celebrity chefs, people making and baking
and demonstrating, and great wine. Anything to do with
the food side of the business is down to Joan, so we usually
get an invite.

The barns is the kind of place that attracts tourists,
yummy mummies, well-preserved grandparents, hard-line
home cooks and lots of gay guys. If you want the latest
gadget or an ingredient that's just been on the TV, the
barns is the place to go, and the staff really know their
stuff; it's a joy to explore and I've never gone there without
buying something. They hold classes in all sorts of things

from bread-making to sugar craft and are always booked solid.

I'd been to their evening events several times, although I hadn't ever expected to go with Max. He showed up at my house bang on time, dressed in jeans and a black T-shirt under a linen jacket and looking just as good dressed down as he did dressed up.

I watched him walk up the path towards the house. My heart did that funny pitter-patter thing that hearts do when you are attracted to someone, accompanied by a little flurry of the clumsiness and self-consciousness that come with the territory. I'm pretty sure it feels just the same whether you're fourteen or eighty.

'All ready?' he asked as I opened the door.

'Yes, Sir,' I said.

'Good. You look very nice,' he said, looking me up and down. 'I thought we'd go in my car again, if you don't mind?' He embraced me and kissed me on both cheeks.

'No, that's fine, Sir,' I said, but I was a bit taken aback. No kinky stuff? No whipping? No nipple clamps? No promise of things to come? To be honest, I was a bit disappointed.

'I didn't think you did vanilla, Sir.'

Max grinned. 'I don't,' he said, as I picked up my bag and locked up.

Max opened the car door for me. He had emailed me instructions to wear a dress for our evening out – a dress, stockings and suspenders, along with the necklace, which I now wore all the time – and as we were going to be with my friends he had said that I could wear a bra and knickers.

I wasn't quite sure what I had expected, but I wasn't complaining. I wondered what the others would make of him.

As we pulled away from the kerb, Max said, 'It's great that you and your friends look out for each other.'

I nodded.

'And I appreciate your concerns about this being vanilla, Sarah, but what you need to understand is that the fundamental rules don't change just because we're with them. Or if we're anywhere else, come to that.'

'I have to call you Sir?' I said incredulously.

Max grinned. 'No, not while we're in your friends' company. Tonight Max will be just fine.'

'What do you mean, then, Sir?'

'Your status remains unchanged, Sarah. The dynamics of this are always the same: you're still my sub wherever we are, whatever you're doing, whether you're with me or not. And if you break the rules, you will be punished. Remember that.'

I glanced across at him. His expression was fixed and he kept his eyes on the road. Part of me got a thrill from what he was saying. I was enjoying the things we had been doing and what we were building between us – and I realized that there was also part of me that was relieved. I didn't want the BDSM element to be switched on and off. I liked the fact that as far as he was concerned it was always there, and that when I was with him there were rules. It made me feel safe, which came as something of a revelation.

'Do you have any questions?' he asked.

'When we're with my friends, are you expecting me to be quiet or anything or be –' I struggled to find the words to describe what I meant, and ended up saying, 'you know, more *slavey*, Sir?'

Max laughed. 'Good God, no. Are you serious? What the hell would your friends think? No, of course not. I want them to see that you're OK, not have me arrested. No, just be yourself. I like who you are; I don't want you to try and be something else. Yes, there are rules of engagement when we're together, but you'll get used to them, until they come naturally wherever we are, but there's no challenge training a doormat. A good Dom should help you to become more of who you are, not less – I'm a sadist, not a psychopath. Now, tell me where we have to go.'

Joan's shop is about twenty minutes' drive away from where I live. Once we got within half a mile or so of it, we joined a steady stream of traffic making its way towards the barns.

The barns are arranged in a squared U-shape around a large gravel courtyard, which has chairs and tables and quite big trees in urns. Tonight the trees were strung with fairy lights. The entrance was fronted by an open-sided marquee full of stalls and stands, and was decked with bunting. A jazz band was playing. Off to one side the barbecue was all fired up, and a chef from *Ready Steady Cook* was getting ready to do something interesting with two bags of ingredients garnered from the barns' deli. Hanging out by the 'this season's new wine' tasting table I could see Helen, Gabbie and Joan, who though technically at work was obviously not planning to miss out on meeting my new man. I spotted them watching Max and me from the minute we got out of the car. They'd obviously deliberately picked their spot to give them an all-round view.

We had arrived fairly early, but if Max was rattled by the way the three of them tracked our progress he certainly didn't show it – and didn't so much as hesitate as we headed towards them.

As I made the introductions, Joan whispered, 'Shaun's here.' Presumably this was in case I felt the need to change horses halfway through the evening. Gabbie held out a hand. Max grasped it firmly and, looking her straight in the eyes, said, 'So what exactly is it that you want to know?'

Gabbie laughed. 'Everything, obviously,' she replied. 'Helen will be taking notes.'

As an opener it was perfect and a sign of things to come. Max chatted to all of them, made them laugh, explored the stalls with us, tried cheeses and chutneys, bought ice creams all round, giggled with the rest of us when Helen won a bright pink very phallic-looking hand blender, and was generally fabulous. Any concerns I'd had about him mixing with the girls rapidly evaporated. He was great company, funny, not over-familiar, chatty, asked all the right questions – perfect.

A while later we were standing in the queue for the barbecue with the others, deciding what to have from the menu, which was written on a giant blackboard behind the grills.

'What are you going to have?' I asked him, scanning down the list. Ostrich burger? Chilli prawns? Wild boar burgers?'

Max smiled and leaned in close so that none of the others could hear him. 'What I'm going to have is you taking your knickers off and then bringing them back to me,' he said. 'And don't be long. I'll be timing you. You'll be punished if you take too long. One stroke for every minute.'

I stared at Max as he moved along with the queue, smiling at my friends and picking up plates and cutlery for both of us from the service table.

'If you want to go, you'd better go now. We're nearly at the front of the queue,' he said brightly, as if we had been mid-conversation – and whatever it was had been my idea. 'And don't worry, I'll get your food.'

While we were out in the company of my friends it was easy to forget that inside the urbane affable man was a man whose greatest pleasure came from dominating his women, whipping them and tying them up – and it took me by surprise how very quickly he changed from one to the other. But I can't deny that it was exciting too.

I turned and hurried across the gravel.

'Where are you going?' asked Gabbie, breaking ranks.

'I just need to pop to the loo,' I said.

'Oh good, me too. Hold on, I'll come with you,' she said, turning to hand Helen her plate and tell Helen, Joan and Max what she wanted from the menu. She couldn't make her mind up. All the time she was speaking, Max's gaze was on me. He glanced fleetingly at his watch. He was keeping track of the minutes. I was wondering exactly how long I'd got and what my punishment might be if I over-ran. A little thread of adrenaline kicked in: pain and pleasure, wasn't that what Max promised me? That wherever we were it was never going to be vanilla: however innocent it looked from the outside, the game was always on.

As we walked across the gravel, Gabbie slipped her arm through mine and pulled me in tightly up against her. 'Well, well, well, Ms K, no wonder you've been hiding Max away. Are there any more at home like him?' she teased. 'How long have you two been seeing each other?' She looked at me and grinned. 'Oh, come off it, spill the beans, Sarah. He's fabulous. It's not like you to be so tight-lipped. 'Fess up. I want to know every last sordid detail. Look at you, all glowing and gorgeous. You don't need to be a genius to see you've got it bad, and I'm not surprised. So ...' She paused, her eyes bright with amusement. 'What's he like in the sack?'

Straight to the point, our Gabbie.

'Inventive,' I said, as I slipped into the toilet cubicle in front of her.

'Lucky, lucky girl,' she said, through the closed door, as I was inside standing on one leg trying to take my knickers off, roll them up and put them in my handbag without falling over or dropping them onto the floor of the cubicle.

'Did you say he'd got a brother?' she called.

I laughed. 'No, or at least not that I know of.'

'Damn. Shame about that. I might have to go and give Shaun the once-over.'

'Be my guest,' I said, pressing the flush.

Given that I'd been allowed to keep my underwear on for this evening's trip out, I'd worn one of my favourite dresses. It's retro, a classic *Mad Men* shirtwaister with buttons all the way down the front, in navy with white spots, wide shoulders, tight nipped-in belted waist and a floaty bias-cut skirt. It's the perfect shape for me – but it certainly isn't the ideal dress to wear without knickers. One stray gust of wind and I'd be revealing a lot more than my pudgy white thighs. The way it felt, actually, I might as well have been stark naked as we headed back to find Max and the others – and my guess is that that was the whole point. Gabbie was still talking, but to be perfectly honest my mind wasn't on the conversation.

'Are you listening to me?' snapped Gabbie. She'd obviously noticed too.

'Sorry?'

'I was just saying that I wanted to go and take a look at the cupcakes over there. They've got a woman doing a demonstration. They're absolutely amazing. Have you seen them?'

'No –' I began.

'Come on, let's go and have a quick look,' said Gabbie, slipping her arm back through mine. 'They'll be ages before they get to the front of the queue. And I want to hear all about Max.'

'I'd rather go back,' I protested, glancing back towards the others.

Gabbie stared at me. 'What, and miss out on free cake? Are you serious? It's not like you, sweetie. Surely he won't miss you for five minutes? Or are you worried he'll run off with Helen?'

'No, of course not,' I blustered. I took another look back towards the barbecue, convinced that Max would be watching my progress and counting the minutes.

Gabbie had taken my reply as a green light and was steering me towards a long table where a woman was rolling out pastel-coloured icing and creating intricate flowers with which to decorate a row of tiny cakes. There was a plate of samples to try in the shape of spring flowers, butterflies and ladybirds.

Nothing could have been a greater contrast to where my mind was. What was my punishment if I over-ran the allotted time? What had Max got planned? How long had I got?

At the other end of the counter the cake-maker's assistants were selling the fruits of her labours, along with a selection of tools and cutters with which to make the cakes and their decorations. Gabbie wanted an excuse to buy some. There was a queue. I was getting twitchy.

'I'll get us some for dessert, shall I?' Gabbie was saying as the queue shuffled forward. 'And I'd quite like a box to take home. What do you fancy?' She rolled her eyes as I was about to speak. 'Don't tell me, *Max* ...'

Groaning inwardly I waited, feeling Max's eyes on me while Gabbie deliberated. Lemon or vanilla? Carrot cupcake or toffee?

'We ought to get back,' I pressed. Yes, I could easily have gone back on my own but it made me look a bit clingy, as if I couldn't bear to be away from him, and there was part of me that liked the fact I was breaking the rules, anticipating what the punishment might be.

'Are those ones lemon too?' Gabbie was asking the girl with the cake tongs.

Watching the cake-maker – who was busily pressing a little hinged cutter into raspberry-pink icing – made me think about nipple clamps. I shivered.

'Hurry up,' I hissed.

Gabbie glanced over her shoulder. 'For goodness' sake, they're not even at the front of the queue yet,' she said. 'Relax.'

Easier said than done. I glanced down nervously at my dress, wondering if any of the buttons were loose. Would they gape when I sat down? Just how see-through was this fabric?

When we finally did head over to find the others, Helen and Joan were sitting at one of the picnic benches by the bar, eating and deep in conversation with Max. They didn't give me a second look as I slipped into the seat opposite them, but Max did.

'We got spiced chicken and salad, or beef with onions and salad,' Helen said.

'God, those look fabulous,' said Gabbie, settling in with her boxes of cupcakes and helping herself to a burger from a stack on the plate in the centre of the table. 'I'm famished. We got some cakes for dessert.' She took a big bite out of her burger and purred. 'Wow, that's amazing.'

'Local beef,' Joan was saying. 'We have them made by our butcher.'

Meanwhile, Max smiled at me and held out his hand. I had expected the handover of my underwear to be discreet. I should have known better. I slipped my hand into my bag and pulled out my panties. Max's smile widened as I reached across the table towards him. 'Thank you,' he said.

'Oh great, have you got some tissues?' said Gabbie, through a mouthful of burger. 'Can I have one?'

I reddened, as for one heart-stopping moment I thought Max was going to give her my underwear, but I was saved by Helen, who pointed to the table. 'There you go. I brought a whole stack of napkins over,' she said. 'Help yourself.'

Max, meanwhile, pressed my knickers to his nose and breathed in. I felt my colour deepen.

'Are you enjoying it?' asked Joan, oblivious.

Max nodded. His eyes never left mine. 'Very much so,' he said. 'I'm really looking forward to exploring the rest of it.'

I squirmed, embarrassed, self-conscious, yet at the same time feeling a little flutter of anticipation low down in my belly. As I watched, he wiped his lips and kissed the fabric before tucking it away into his pocket.

'So,' said Gabbie, 'how did you two meet?'

I was about to answer when Max said, 'Online, but come on, Gabbie, I'm sure that you already knew that.'

'True, but I just wondered which site? I'm curious, that's all. I might want to sign up and see what they can do for me.'

I stared at her. Was she flirting with him?

Max took a bite of his burger. 'Sarah can give you the address, if you like. It was one of those kinky sites, whips and chains.'

Gabbie threw back her head and laughed. 'Oh yeah, right,' she said. 'I can believe that. Mind you, I'm tempted to look if they're all like you.'

'You should try it,' he said.

'I just might do that,' she said.

I slapped her with a fork. 'Behave.'

'What? What's the problem?' Gabbie protested. 'I was only asking.'

'Well, don't. How many glasses of wine have you had?'

'Just one, and besides you know how it is: there's been a bit of a drought this year –'

'Don't ask Max to fix you up with a man,' I warned.

'Why don't you get Joan to introduce you to Shaun, Gabbie?' asked Max, full of mischief. 'He sounds like he's worth a shot.'

I stared at him, eyes wide.

'For Sarah, maybe, but not me. He's lovely, apparently,' said Gabbie. 'I reckon I need someone a bit more meaty than lovely. I put men off – too assertive.'

I stared at Max. 'How do you know about Shaun?'

'Joan told me,' he said, nodding across the table.

Joan grinned self-consciously and turned her attention back to her food.

'Oh, it's fine,' said Max, with good humour. 'I think always having a man in reserve is a great idea.'

'I'll remember that,' I said, determined not to be fazed by him.

After we'd eaten, Joan needed to go back to help out, so Max, Helen, Gabbie and I wandered over to where the celebrity chef was warming up his wok. Quite a crowd had gathered in front of the dais to watch the demonstration.

Max stood behind me, his hands resting easily on my waist. I liked the way it felt. He leaned in closer and kissed my neck. As the chef kicked off his presentation, one hand crept down towards my hip and then down over my buttock in long, gently circling strokes. He was making me very aware of being knickerless.

On stage the chef was cutting and chopping with breathtaking skill, although it was hard to concentrate on the cooking.

Max leaned in close and whispered, 'Eleven minutes.' I glanced up at him. I knew exactly what he meant.

'Eleven?' I repeated.

He nodded. 'That's what I said. You questioning me?'

I shook my head, feeling my heart rate quicken. I realized that while part of me was dreading the punishment, another part could hardly wait. Max ran a finger up my spine. 'I'm going to enjoy spanking you so much,' he whispered.

Up on the dais the chef was busy swapping wisecracks with the audience. As more and more people gathered around to watch, Max moved closer still, till his whole body was pressed up against mine.

'I've brought my riding crop with me,' he said in an undertone. I shivered.

Alongside me Gabbie looked across with a question in her expression. 'You OK?' she mouthed. I nodded.

Max's hands circled my waist, while up on stage the chef tipped the pan he was using forward into the gas flame and the ingredients caught light, flambéing the contents. As the crowd gasped with delight, Max slid his hand down over my stomach and for the briefest of instants his fingers slipped between the buttons of my dress and brushed over the rise of my sex. His touch was as fleeting as it was deliberate and sent a great ripple of desire through me.

'You smell fabulous,' he whispered. 'And I love the fact you're naked under your dress. Do you know how much I want you?'

My legs turned to jelly.

As the demonstration came to an end the chef and the barn staff handed round tiny portions of the food for every-one to try. The chef was selling his latest book, the shop was selling the ingredients, and on the table to one side of the dais was a huge hamper, which was being raffled off, along with a weekend cookery course.

'We should get some tickets,' said Gabbie to the rest of us, as the demo came to a close. We shuffled our way to the front and Max bought two – one for me and one for him – and then took both tickets to fill in the address stubs, before handing one over to me.

'Can you just check yours?' he said casually, handing me a pen.

I nodded. Max had taken his time, but my address wasn't complicated. He handed me the ticket, along with

a small sheet of paper. I checked the raffle ticket, tore off
the stub to put into the tombola and then looked at the
sheet of paper. On it was stuck a Post-it note, which
read:

ADDENDUM

Further to our recent discussions I agree to let my
Master use me sexually in any way he chooses.
  My Master has been looking forward to fucking
me since the day we first met.
  Signed:

I looked up at Max, feeling myself blush and a great rush
of heat rippling through me.

Max grinned. 'You might like to sign that,' he said,
indicating the pen with a nod of his head.

'What's taking you two so much time?' said
Gabbie, who had already bought her tickets and sorted
out the stubs. She glanced across at me as I covered
the Post-it and signed the additional clause to our
contract.

'You don't have to fill anything in on that bit,' she said
incredulously. 'You just need to write your address on the
stub.' As she spoke she leaned over, making as if to take
the ticket and the slip of paper, but Max was too quick for
her.

'I'll keep that for you if you like, Sarah,' he said, sliding
the piece of paper out from between my fingers and into
his inside pocket.

Gabbie looked at me and frowned. I knew that she guessed something was going on but I wasn't going to say anything.

Instead, I smiled at her and then at Max. 'That sounds like a good idea. Keep it safe,' I said casually.

He made a show of glancing down at his watch. 'Unfortunately we have to be going soon,' he said. 'I've got something special planned for Sarah tonight.' And with that he took my hand.

Gabbie raised her eyebrows. 'Lucky girl,' she purred, winking at me. If only she knew.

Before we left, Max and I did the rounds and said our goodbyes to Helen and Joan, who were as impressed with Max as Gabbie was.

It was a lovely evening. The sky had darkened to a lush indigo and stars were shining like spilt rhinestones. As we walked back along the drive, I could hear the jazz band on the breeze. I felt really happy, and totally at ease with myself and what was going on. Whatever it was that Max had planned, I was content to let him lead the way. It was a heady sensation, handing your wellbeing over to someone else. I was used to looking after myself, so there was something exquisite in choosing to let go a little and switch off the control freakery.

As we got back to the car park, Max caught hold of me and, spinning me around, pinned me up against the car and slid his hand between my legs, gathering up the fabric of my dress, his fingers seeking out the soft moist folds of my sex, his fingers pressed inside me, brushing my clitoris, exploring and stroking. His touch took my breath away. His fingers were rough and proprietorial, and set me on fire.

'Well,' he said, looking me straight in the eye, 'I think that went well, don't you? And you are so very wet ...' I looked away, self-conscious, embarrassed and perturbed by just how much I wanted him.

'Do you think I passed inspection?' he asked, leaning around me to open the car door.

'Yes, Sir,' I said.

'You don't want to go back and see how Shaun shapes up, then?'

I shook my head.

'Good. Now let's get out of here. I've got a little treat planned for you.' He grinned. 'Actually eleven little treats.'

Chapter Fifteen

'I always want to know the things one shouldn't do.'
'So as to do them?' asked her aunt.
'So as to choose,' said Isabel.
Henry James

By the time we reached our destination it was completely dark. Max guided the car off the main road, taking us down mile after mile of winding country lanes before finally heading on to a narrow track. We bumped down off the tarmac. Max slowed the car to a crawl as we made our way between the ruts where a green lane wound its way in and out between stands of mature trees. I had no idea where we were. Eventually, after what seemed like an age, we reached a small clearing that was completely surrounded by silver birches, their stems glowing an eerie white in the gloom. Max cut the engine.

We sat for a few seconds without speaking. It was uncannily quiet in the woods, the only sound the gentle tick, tick, ticking of the engine as it cooled.

After a second or two, Max climbed out of the car, came round to my side and opened the door.

'Out,' he said, offering me his hand. 'Leave your bag.'

I looked up at him nervously. We were miles from anywhere. I couldn't see a light or a house for miles.

Max's expression hardened. 'Now,' he said crisply. There was no threat in his voice, just an assumption that I should and would do exactly as I was told.

I took his hand and clambered out onto the damp, uneven grass. Moonlight and stars bathed the clearing in a soft, silvery glow. My night vision isn't great, so it took a while for my eyes to adjust to the gloom and get my bearings.

Max took his holdall and a blanket from the boot, put my handbag in the boot in their place and locked the car before leading me along a narrow trail between the trees that led deeper into the woods. His stride was measured and confident, mine much less so. I was wearing high-heeled sandals. OK, not that high, but not designed with cross-country hiking in mind. After a couple of hundred yards the trail broadened out and I finally settled into step with him, trying hard not to stumble on the tussocks and ruts.

'You OK?' Max asked.

'Just about,' I said, slapping my arm, sure that I had been bitten by a nasty little flying beastie. 'Where is this, Sir?'

I must have sounded overly anxious, because Max turned to look at me when he replied. 'It's a piece of woodland owned by some friends of mine.'

'And do they know we're here?'

He grinned. 'I might have mentioned to them that I'd be out this way over this weekend.'

I looked back over my shoulder, wondering if he had mentioned to them that he would be showing up in the middle of the night.

Finally we came to a second clearing, divided by a fallen tree and a row of stumps, which had been cut low and painted white so that they looked like stepping stones. I could hear running water from a stream, and close to the stumps were a table and benches, with a barbecue not far away. Looking round, I wondered momentarily if we were going to have a picnic.

I imagine in daylight the clearing was a fabulous spot, but in moonlight while it was still quite beautiful there was something slightly eerie and unsettling about it too. I shivered as Max dropped his bag onto one of the benches and spread the blanket over the table.

'Take off your dress,' he said over his shoulder without so much as a glance in my direction. He took a Maglite out of his pocket and, holding it between his teeth, began to unpack the bag.

'Are you serious? What if someone sees us, Sir?' I said, looking round. Which was a crazy idea: unless Max's friends planned to show up or had night-vision goggles we couldn't have been further from civilization if we'd taken a coracle. I watched Max unpack his bag, the toys, the crop and a blanket, but I didn't move.

'Unless of course you'd like me to rip your dress off you,' he said, without looking up. 'Would you prefer that? I'm very happy to oblige.' Very slowly he turned towards me, eyes glittering in the moonlight.

I knew that it wasn't an idle threat, and that all I had to do was say the word and Max would be there. I glanced down. It was my favourite dress. For a moment or two I toyed with the idea of him chasing me through the woods before ravishing me down among the bracken. Realistically the chances were that I'd trip and fall over and probably break something, and besides I'd bought this dress years ago and there was no way I'd ever get another one like it, however much I loved it.

'Well?' pressed Max. 'What is it to be?'

I began to undo the buttons of my dress, slowly, nervously glancing left and right in case we were being watched – although by what or whom exactly I'm not sure.

Max held out a hand to take the dress from me. I swallowed hard, delaying the moment. He waited patiently. Carefully I slipped it off my shoulders and down over my arms, before finally handing it over. There is something deeply unsettling both about being watched and about undressing outdoors. Other than awkward self-conscious moments undressing on the beach, I'd never been naked outside before. The breeze caressed my skin, making me tingle all over. The sensation was electrifying. I felt a rush of adrenaline, quickening my pulse. Around me I could hear the sounds of the woods; an owl hooted right on cue, animals were moving around in the undergrowth and I could hear the wind skittering through the leaves.

'And your bra as well,' Max said.

I did as I was told, despite feeling incredibly vulnerable, naked now except for my stockings, suspenders and shoes. The night air was cool and raised goosebumps on my skin; my nipples stiffened in the night breeze.

'I'm cold,' I said.

'Won't be for long,' he said, running the torchlight over my body, the white-blue beam as cool and invasive as his fingertips. 'Now give me your hands,' he said.

I held them out in front of me, dazzled by the torch-light, as he fastened a leather cuff onto each wrist in turn, each with a D ring set into it. An odd state of calm settled over me as I watched him buckling them up. It was a strange state of mind that submission had led me into. I wondered if this was how rabbits feel when they are caught in the headlights of a car. It felt like an easy, waking sleep; still, calm – almost meditative. I waited, compliant and passive, as Max threw a rope up over a branch on one of the trees on the edge of the clearing and then came back to lead me towards it.

'Put your hands out now,' he said. There was a sliding bolt clip, like the kind of thing you get on a dog lead, fixed into the rope, which he fastened to the D rings on my cuffs, and then he very gently hauled the rope up over the branch until I was at full stretch and standing on tiptoe. As soon as he was happy with my position, he tied off the rope.

The stretch made me gasp. The only respite was to pull one way or the other and take the rope with me, taking one foot completely off the ground and standing on the other foot, but even then it wasn't quite flat on the floor. As I tried to find the most comfortable position the torch went out, and for a moment or two I couldn't see anything. Very gradually my eyes readjusted.

In the light from the moon Max gave me time to settle. He ran a hand over my back: his touch was calming, a physical reassurance that everything was OK and that he was there, that he was in control of what was going on, and of me, and that this was exactly what he wanted to happen. All was well. As I hung there in silence, waiting for whatever was going to happen next, the breeze picked up, stirring the leaves around my feet. I felt more than naked as the wind chilled me.

With slow deliberation Max ran his hands over my arms and shoulders, as if savouring the moment and checking that I was hanging properly; then he buried his face in the crook of my neck, alternately biting and kissing, cupping my breasts as he did. His hands were warm on my cold skin. He was working his way down over my waist and hips and buttocks, exploring without hindrance, nipping and teasing, stroking and touching. Each brush of his fingertips, tongue, lips and teeth lit little trails of tinder through my body, making me gasp and shiver and sigh, his caress sensitizing every last inch of me.

Circling me, Max drew first one breast and then the other into his mouth, sucking hard at my nipples, biting down, squeezing the tender flesh. My excitement grew with each caress, with each little shard of pleasure and pain, and my reluctance to be naked in the great outdoors receded with every passing second.

Max moved lower, his lips and tongue seeking out the sensitive places, exploring my chilled flesh, kissing my belly, the curve of my hip, the base of my spine, my thighs, the backs of my knees. All of my body, all of me at that moment, belonged to Max; there was nowhere that he couldn't touch or explore, no place that was off-limits. As his fingers and tongue worked their magic, my mind and body were ablaze with sensation.

Standing up, he slid his hand between my legs, opening me, his fingers eager to find their way inside me. This time I knew that I was wet. I moaned desperately at his touch and pressed my body against him, hungry for more. Then I started to feel nipping – and realized he was putting little clips on my skin, under my arms, on the swell of my breast, on the skin over my hips and ribs, and on each ear lobe, and the clips were connected by a long white cord. The pressure was not unpleasant but made me aware of parts of my body I was usually oblivious to.

'Left-hand or right-hand pocket?' he asked. 'You can choose what comes next.'

'What?' I gasped. I was not really in any sort of state to take part in a pop quiz.

'That's "What, Sir". Just answer the question, Sarah. It's very simple. Left or right?'

I found myself trying to work out what Max was really asking me – quite obviously impossible when there were no clues, but I found myself trying anyway. I was feeling drunk on adrenaline, desire and expectation.

'I'm waiting,' Max said.

'Left,' I said.

'Good choice.' He stood far enough away so that I could see him, now that my eyes had become accustomed to the strange grey metallic moonlight, and pulled something out from his pocket. I tried to focus on it, screwing up my eyes to help me understand what I was seeing. There was a flash of what I thought was bright pink and something much darker, black maybe. From the colour and the shapes my brain joined the dots: it was a ball gag. My eyes widened. Max held it up for me to admire. 'Left it is,' he said.

'How can I say the safe word with a gag in, Sir?' I protested before he could fasten it into place.

'If you clench and unclench your hands I'll know something is wrong and I'll stop. And don't worry: I'll be watching you all the time. Now open your mouth.'

I resisted for an instant, pressing my lips together, defiantly meeting his gaze. I could see the amusement in his eyes and something I could only interpret as tenderness. He waited.

'Open your mouth,' he repeated. This time I did as I was told. The ball was a little larger than a ping-pong ball and made of dense resin. It tasted vaguely chemical. I could either let it sit in my mouth or push it forward with my tongue and lips and hold it between my teeth. I could also still make a noise. Max watched me experimenting.

'Eleven minutes,' he said.

I knew exactly what he meant. 'Oh, and an additional one minute for speaking without permission and another for a missing Sir. Which makes thirteen in all, but as I'm feeling generous we'll call it a round dozen, shall we?' As he was talking Max took something else from his other pocket. It took me seconds to realize that it was a blindfold, but it was too late to protest or do anything about it as he slipped it over my head. I was stunned.

Naked, gagged, blindfolded, nipped by tiny clips and hanging from a tree in the middle of woods miles from anywhere is probably a little bit outside most people's comfort zone, and when I think about it rationally the same is true of me, except there was a part of me that loved it – that loves it. Here I felt so alive, full of sensations, every cell alight with expectation and something indefinable and compelling that glowed white hot in every molecule. Here all the things that I am came together and joined up.

As I was hanging there, in my mind I replayed the position of the D rings and the hook arrangement. I was not locked to anything and if I pulled the rope down hard over the branch I was more or less certain I could free myself. There is never a scenario that I've been involved in, in BDSM, however involved I am, however excited, where I haven't planned my escape if things go wrong, and I've refused point blank to play if I can't see a way of getting out. I trusted Max, but more than that I trusted myself – something that BDSM has made me more conscious of.

I wait. I ease my weight from foot to foot. I can hear Max moving around. I am waiting, but nothing prepares me for the hot, slicing explosion of the pain across my back. I shriek and buck against the cuffs as the sensation suffuses every nerve ending, flooding through every part of me and filling my head with stars. The cry is muffled and deadened by the ball gag. It is different from the cane in subtle ways, oddly more bearable but no less painful.

'I won't ask you to count,' Max says.

There is nothing inherently good about this; it's hard to explain unless you are attracted to it – there is nothing good about being whipped or flogged or caned. It hurts.

But what *is* good is the place it takes me to, which I can't reach any other way. I love it and I hate it. I relish the fight, the challenge of it – and when I am not being tied or whipped I fondly imagine that when Max beats me next time somehow I will like it for itself – that I will hang on, hang tough, fight the sensations, be strong enough to deal with it. That's nonsense. It always hurts, though it is true that over time you grow to be able to tolerate more. But I am never immune to the pain. I always hate it and I know as the second blow cracks across my backside that I will never, ever be ready for the pain. The paradox of wanting something and hating something is not lost on me.

I hear myself crying and sobbing, begging him to stop, struggling against my restraints, losing myself in the blizzard of the feelings.

I cry out, twisting under the rope, tears rolling down my face, and at the same time I feel myself on the abyss, peering down into a place that only pain can take me to.

Max hits me again. I swing round so that this time the crop catches the underside of my breasts, catching one of the plastic clips. A shriek explodes deep down in my throat. I can stop this any time I want. I know the signal. I know how to make it stop, but I don't. Some part of my brain tries to occupy itself counting the strokes.

After four Max leans in close to me. His touch on my face is as gentle as that of any lover that I've ever had. 'Do you want me to stop?' he asks.

I hesitate; this is my get-out-of-jail-free card. I know that he won't be upset or angry that I've cried off; I know that's not how this works. He will stop if I want to. He stopped before; he will be happy to stop again.

'Tell me to stop,' he says, his breath soft on my face. 'Tell me.'

I shake my head.

He doesn't ask me again. Instead I gasp at the pain as the next stroke hits home, cracking across my buttocks, hard and hot, and as it echoes through me I let go. I am a mess. Tears are streaming down my face. My throat is sore and dry from shrieking and sobbing and begging Max to stop, knowing full well that he won't unless I give him the signal. And I won't do that. I have no idea how many times Max hits me. He said twelve but I'm not counting.

And then it is over. I am completely turned inside out, every inch of me tingling, skinned, wired and alive. After twelve strokes Max's strong gentle hands unfasten my wrists and take my weight, unfasten the ball gag and hold me tightly against him. His fingers pull away the clips.

Still unable to see because of the mask, I curl up against his chest and let him hold me tightly into his body while he makes noises of comfort and pride, and all the while he strokes my hair. And yes, this is madness, yet as I lean into his strong, muscular body, hot now from the exertion of punishing me, I love being there; I love the sensation of being held by him, and I can sense his excitement and mine. Held tightly in his arms, I can hear his racing heart and there is nowhere else I would rather be. How do you work this out and make sense of it? I've come to the conclusion that Max is right: you can't, and you would drive yourself crazy trying.

As I start to recover, Max turns me around and snaps the cuffs together behind my back, which confirms what I suspected – the beating is just the opening act in tonight's proceedings.

As he turns me back towards him I hear the sound of a zipper and don't protest as he guides me towards the ground. Sinking to my knees among the leaf mould and the cones, finally after all the weeks we have been playing together, I take his cock in my mouth. Unsurprisingly he is rock hard, circumcised, smooth and sleek, thick and silky to the touch. I close my lips around him and take him deeper, trying to keep my balance, trying to give him as much pleasure as he has given me.

I work my tongue up the shaft, under the head, sucking and licking him, lips working around the girth, and above me I hear him sighing with pleasure as my lips close tightly around him, and I take him as deep as I can, struggling to suppress the gag reflex, and I sigh too as finally we move whatever this is that we have on to another level.

I move my head, working up and down the shaft. I am eager to take him to the brink. I try everything I can to make him come, everything I've read, every trick and every subtle touch. I want to give him pleasure and for once, I suppose, to be in control. I want to show him what he has shown me.

This is crazy. Fellatio really isn't my thing, as other men will attest, but tonight it is all I want to do. I lean into him, sinking into the moment, enjoying him, enjoying the sensation I have of both submission – of kneeling at his feet – and power as I bring him closer and closer to orgasm. He tangles his fingers in my hair, pulling me backwards and forwards against his engorged cock, fucking my mouth, and as his excitement builds I feel mine echoing it.

Max's breathing is faster now, his movements ragged, and I think that he is almost there – and then, just as the thought fills my head, he pulls away, gasping, denying me my prize.

I feel robbed and wail in protest. Max pulls me to my feet and, unfastening my cuffs, picks me up and lifts me up onto the picnic table, which he has covered with a blanket. I'm gasping for more now.

He pulls off my mask and grins down at me, eyes alight with desire and hunger. 'You're ready for this?'

I nod, almost afraid to speak in case he denies me yet again.

Max smiles wolfishly. 'I'll forgive you for that this time. God, I want to fuck you so much, Sarah.'

The words make me shiver with delight. He couldn't want me any more than I want him.

He spreads my legs. We've discussed safe sex – is there any other kind? He takes a foil packet from his jacket pocket, opens it and rolls a condom down over his raging erection. My mouth is watering. I want to feel him inside me. Then he brushes the head of his cock between the lips of my sex, and then again. It is the sweetest torture. I want him in me. I want him to fuck me now, to fuck me hard. I look up into his eyes. His jaw is set, his expression determined and focused, and as our eyes meet I groan, trying to lift myself up to take him inside me.

Max grins. 'Greedy. You have to ask me,' he said. 'I want to hear you beg.'

Even now he is the one in control.

'Please,' I whisper.

'Please what?'

'Please, Sir, fuck me.'

'Again.'

'Please, Sir, *fuck me.*'

Oh and he did. The words had barely faded on my lips before Max drove deep into me, taking my breath away. My body opened for him, his arms sliding under my thighs so that he could pull himself deeper still. My sex, warm, wet and eager, closed around him like a clenched fist, his cock filling me to the brim, making me gasp, making me sob, making me cry out for more. I cried out in a mixture of delight and breathless excitement as he found his rhythm. He pressed me back onto the table, each thrust building on the last, driving away every rational thought. My body moved instinctively with his, matching him stroke for stroke, reaching up towards him, bringing us both closer and closer to the brink, and then he said, 'Touch yourself, Sarah. I want to watch you.'

And this time I didn't resist. As my fingers found my clitoris I heard Max groan with pleasure and renew his efforts. The combination was electric: his body moving up against mine, my fingers, his cock. I was drowning, lost in the heat of it – my body arched up to meet his, my fingers working, trapped between his torso and mine. I could feel the pleasure building and building; I felt my sex tighten rhythmically around him. As he pushed into me, I felt his cock pulse deep inside, and it was enough. Gasping, I tumbled headlong with him into the abyss, lost in the sensations and the release, our thrusts ragged and frantic now, both of us crying out as waves of pleasure washed over us.

Then finally it was over. Max collapsed down onto me, his body hot, heavy and spent. He was gasping to catch his breath. We both lay still, wrapped around each other. Then very gently Max pulled away and rolled over onto the table alongside me. I groaned at the loss, feeling totally exposed and utterly naked. Max and I had waited so long to get to this point, but it had been worth the wait. I was full of tears and joy. I couldn't remember a time when sex had been so totally all-consuming, nor how long it was since I had shared a moment like this with someone I truly cared about.

I was cold and breathless, my stockings were ruined, my back was rubbed raw from the beating and from moving wildly up against the table. Max helped me to sit up and handed me my dress.

'No underwear,' he said, and then added, 'Before you put your dress on I want to take a look at your back.'

I stared at him. *Really?*

He pulled out the Maglite from his pocket. 'Here,' he said, patting the end of the table. 'Now,' he said more forcefully. I did as I was told.

I felt strangely self-conscious as Max gently turned me this way and that so that he could examine the marks on my back. He reached down into the holdall he'd brought with him from the car and produced a tub of antiseptic wipes. I laughed. He didn't.

'Stay still. You've got a couple of nasty scratches that I want to clean up.'

'I'll be fine,' I said, wriggling away from him and getting to my feet.

'Sit,' Max snapped. 'I'm going to clean these up. I take care of my property – it's in the contract. Remember?'

The wipes were icy cold and made the grazes and raised welts sting like crazy. I whimpered.

This time it was Max who laughed. 'Don't be such a baby,' he said, bending down to kiss the sore spots. 'I've got something in my bag for your bruises.'

'I haven't got any bruises,' I said, trying to peer over my shoulder.

He took a tube out of the bag and gently rubbed cream into my skin. 'You will have in the morning,' he said.

I winced as the antiseptic went to work.

As I pulled my dress back on I thought about how my life had been changed by meeting Max. He was right: vanilla sex was unlikely ever to be this exciting. As we slowly walked back to the car through the moonlit woods, Max held my hand and kept me close, and as we got back to where we had parked he leant in close to kiss my hair. It might not be vanilla, it might not be the kind of rela- tionship I was used to or expecting, but it felt fabulous.

Chapter Sixteen

'He in a few minutes ravished this fair creature, or
at least would have ravished her, if she had not, by
a timely compliance, prevented him.'
Henry Fielding

As Max opened the boot so that he could put the holdall
in and I could retrieve my handbag, I noticed a small,
furry, obviously well-loved teddy bear wedged into the
boot lining by one of the wheel arches.

'Yours?' I asked, fishing it out from among the more
usual type of things that lurk in any good sadist's boot:
several lengths of synthetic rope, a couple of metres of
chain and various zippered sports bags.

Max smiled. 'No, but I'm really pleased to see it. He's
Ellie's. I wondered where on earth he had got to. We've
been looking high and low for him.'

We? A little alarm bell sounded somewhere in the back
of my head, although Max, by contrast, was totally relaxed
and sounded neither defensive nor guarded. I handed him
the toy and watched his expression soften as he took it.

'Ellie can't get to sleep without her bear. Abby's been
tearing the place apart looking for it.' The alarm bell rang
just a little louder.

'Abby's at yours?' I asked casually as we got into the car. It didn't quite tally with what he'd told me before about his ex-girlfriend being halfway across the country, but I was also anxious not to sound clingy, needy or paranoid.

'No – no, she just dropped Ellie off in the middle of the week, while she went out with some friends. I've been working from home most of this week, so it's worked out really well.' Max turned, put the bear on the back seat and then fired up the engine.

'I thought Abby lived miles away,' I said, trying hard not to sound like a bunny-boiler.

'She did, but she moved back a couple of weeks ago to be nearer her mum and dad. Makes it easier for Ellie. Abby's working more or less full time now, so Ellie goes to her grandma and granddad's after school. I'm pleased really – it means that I get to see more of Ellie. She's close, but not too close, if you know what I mean.'

'You miss her, don't you?' I asked.

He nodded. 'Who, Ellie? Every day. I wasn't around much when the others were growing up. Having Ellie felt like my second chance.'

'Was Abby a –' For some reason I found it hard to use the word 'submissive' when talking about the mother of his child.

'Sub?' He said it for me.

I nodded.

'Yes, or at least she was when we first met. It's like I said, it's very hard to sustain the dynamic day in day out, and then when we knew Ellie was coming along we made a decision to put that side of our relationship on hold for a while. Abby had a tricky pregnancy.'

'And you can't live without it?'

He shook his head. 'If you're asking if that's why we split up, then the answer's no. We put it on the back burner. We played a little but there were other priorities; we both knew that. The main problem stemmed from the fact that Abby is quite a bit younger than me and we had a fairly adventurous life up until Ellie arrived.'

I waited.

'She got fed up with being at home with a young family and being tied down.' He laughed. 'And not in a good way. We discussed having an au pair but Abby wasn't at all keen on the idea. Anyway, while I was away on a contract she met someone else. Someone local, attentive. To be honest, I didn't see it coming. It felt like history repeating itself.'

'It must have hurt.'

Max nodded. 'It did, and I spent a lot of time thinking about what we could have done differently – to put it right, I suppose. We hadn't planned on having a family together. We travelled a lot until Ellie arrived and then Abby wanted to be settled, so we moved here to be close to her family, but I had to work. She felt neglected and left out.'

'Did you meet her when you were working abroad too?' I knew I was beginning to sound like a police interrogator – you know, the one trying to catch the bad guy out.

'No, Abby's English. We didn't meet till I came back over here. I was just about to change jobs and set up on my own. I'd got all sorts of irons in the fire and was looking for other things to do.

'I wasn't looking for a serious relationship but I wasn't not looking for one either, if you know what I mean. My whole life was changing. I met Abby in a club in London. I'd been playing for a few years, met some great people and had a few relationships, but nothing that serious. I'd just split up with another lass, and was over in the UK for a meeting. I went to a club with friends I'd met through Georgina and they knew her.'

'So a blind date, then?'

Max shook his head. 'No, not really. She just happened to be there when we showed up. As I remember, either her friend or the guy she was seeing hadn't made it, so she tagged along with us for the evening and we got talking, had a few drinks. The people I was with had got a party set for that weekend and asked if Abby wanted to come. She was a bit nervous, but she came anyway and we got together then. She had had a bit of a rough ride ...'

I nodded, wondering how much Max was planning to tell me. I knew that if I asked him he would tell me everything I wanted to know, but for some reason I felt uneasy about prying.

When we got back to mine Max came in for coffee. A first.

'I'd like to thank you for a lovely evening,' he said. Then he laughed. 'I hope your friends approved.'

'Oh, they'll ring,' I said confidently. 'Probably not until Monday now.'

'Because they'll assume I'm staying for the weekend.'

I nodded.

'I will stay,' he said gently. 'But not this weekend. OK?'

We sat on either side of my kitchen table. He smiled at me in the lamplight. I wasn't sure what to say. I wanted him to stay; I wanted to wake up with him in the morning.

'I have to go,' he said, draining the mug.

'Do you?'

He nodded. 'I've got Ellie coming over first thing tomorrow morning and if I stay here I won't want to leave.'

I smiled. 'You think?'

'You don't?' he purred. 'Soon, I promise. There are just some things I need to sort out.'

After Max had gone I cleared away the mugs and went upstairs. I believed him when he said he wanted to stay. My body ached and was covered in dust and leaf mould from the woods. I went into the bathroom and turned on the shower. My back was criss-crossed with bruises and long areas of broken skin. Showering was a nightmare, a sharp reminder of my encounter with Max and our night in the woods, which set me thinking about our first monumental fuck, which made me think about just how much more I wanted.

Chapter Seventeen

'Lust's passion will be served; it demands,
it militates, it tyrannizes.'
Marquis de Sade

I was finding it hard to concentrate on any work. Max had
sent me an email that read:

> On Friday evening you will drive to The – Hotel near –.
> I have reserved a room in the name of Mr and Mrs Smith.
>   You will collect an envelope from reception.
>   Your instructions will be inside.
>   You will wear something obvious, something slutty.
>   You may wear a coat.
>   I will be expecting you at 7.30 p.m.
>   You will not be expected to stay the night.
>   Max

I work from home most of the time and spend long days
in my office alone – if you discount the phone, the dog, the
cat, a pile of paperwork and more books than it can possibly be healthy for one person to own. I was on a tight
deadline to deliver my new book and an even tighter one

to do the edits for the previous one. I'd hit the ground running, but despite my best efforts it was proving hard to keep my mind on the job. Instead I kept going back and re-reading Max's email, enjoying the little flutter of expectation it gave me. And it didn't fade; instead, if anything it got more intense.

At this rate I was going to be totally exhausted by Friday. Max had a natural gift for planting seeds that grew in my imagination. Since we'd met I felt as if I was constantly turned on. Every meeting, every phone call, every text and email had a sexual charge and an erotic subtext, some more overt than others.

He would often send me texts or one-line emails during the course of the day that ensured that he was never far from my mind, and nor were the things he could do to and with me.

It was the sweetest, most delicious torture and one that I was thoroughly enjoying. Max was everything and more that a girl could want from her first Dom. While it might not be helping my work schedule it was doing wonders for my fantasy life, and the weight was just falling off.

I had been wondering if there was a market for the deviant's diet: how to fantasize yourself slim. The downside was that Max had forbidden me from masturbating, so alongside the increased desire was an ever-increasing, aching, all-day-long need – with no release except for the one I knew that he would give me. On the plus side, every time we played together Max made sure I got what I needed: a crashing, all-consuming orgasm – something I

had never been certain of in all the years of vanilla sex –
and sometimes more than one. The downside, or upside
depending on how you looked at it, was that our encounters always left me wanting more, which I suspect was the
whole point. It had also occurred to me that I was impos-
ing the rules on myself: realistically Max would never
know if I was masturbating when he wasn't there, but I
would.

I had already Googled the hotel he'd invited me to,
and sorted out how to get there with an online route
planner.

The hotel was plush, pricy and miles from anywhere,
with a full gym, pool, Jacuzzi and spa, and a fabulous-
looking restaurant. It looked like the perfect place for a
romantic weekend away, although I had to remind myself
that whatever it was that Max and I had it wasn't strictly
romance; it was something else for which I hadn't yet
found a name. Still, it was a pity we weren't staying over.
Or was it just me who wasn't staying over?

As I scrolled through the hotel's website it occurred to
me that what I'd really like was some vanilla time there
with Max so that we could get to know each other better.
Maybe I could persuade him that it was a good idea. When
we talked – and we talked a lot – we had enough in
common to make us a good match and enough that was
different to make it interesting. Had I met Max in any
other way I would have thought that there was a fair
chance our relationship could grow into something altogether bigger and longer lasting. I took a couple of calming breaths and tried to stop my imagination running

away with me. We hadn't met any other way and Max had made it perfectly clear that he didn't do vanilla.

I glanced back at his email. Booking in as Mr and Mrs Smith made me smile. I couldn't help wondering what Max had got in mind; in fact I spent most of the morning letting myself toy with all sorts of possibilities, each more distracting than the last. By lunchtime I'd scoured the website – the beds were huge, canopied creations, and some of the rooms had a four-poster option. I'd always had a fantasy about being strapped between the posts of a bed with soft leather thongs. Had I told Max that? Or was it in one of my books? I looked back at the pile of pages in my in-tray. This was not getting my edits done.

Despite the prospect of playing in a swanky hotel, I had been hoping that we might go back to Max's place over the weekend. He had been to my house on several occasions, and you know by now that I'm nosey. I wanted to see where he lived. You can tell so much about someone by the way they live, what they like, what they value and enjoy. I also understood that with Max's son living with him it was tricky, but it would have been nice to pop in – maybe just have a coffee. It wasn't that I wanted to let either my family or his into what we were doing; coming home to find your father horsewhipping a woman in a leather corset really wasn't on my to-do list. But me meeting Max at his place – that would work, even if I didn't go inside. Maybe I should suggest it to him.

Or maybe I was just looking for things to pick at. The sex was great, the conversation fun, Max was good company and he was only too pleased to tie me up and punish me:

what more could a girl want? The bottom line was that what I wanted was more of him. We saw each other almost every weekend but only ever on a Friday or Saturday, never both, and he still wasn't staying over. I'd be lying if I didn't say I'd also been thinking quite a lot about Abby, Ellie and the teddy bear.

Max had always made it plain that he was still very fond of both his ex-wife and his ex-partner, and that after the blame, the hurt, the chaos and general spite that goes with splitting up he'd managed to find a good place to be in with both of them. He wasn't at all self-conscious about saying how much he had loved them, nor how in a strange way he loved them still.

And yes, I know that I should have been pleased to be with someone who'd negotiated the tricky territory between his exes with such obvious skill. He also seemed to have a good relationship with his children, which was one of the reasons his son was staying with him while he sorted out a job and a flat of his own, and he saw Ellie as often as he could. Yes, all this was commendable – fabulous: he was a good person even when he was whipping the hide off a body.

So why did the teddy bear in the boot make me feel uncomfortable and uneasy? I'd no idea. He certainly didn't come across as or claim to be any kind of goodie two shoes when it came to relationships.

Maybe I was jealous; maybe I'm a naturally suspicious person; maybe I was looking for bad where there was none, trying to pick holes in something that on the face of it appeared to be what I'd been looking for, just so I'd prepare myself for being hurt and let down. Maybe it was just knowing that I was one of many; maybe I'm not as confident and balanced as I like to think; maybe I was being hormonal. But the more I looked at my own emotional discomfort, the less sense it made.

I loved my own children and although I wouldn't say I was on amicable terms with my ex yet, we could just about now talk to each other without going over the same old ground, and I could see a time coming when we would be able to talk like reasonable people – well, I would talk like one, anyway. So what was it about Max and his exes that was bugging me? I wished I knew.

Halfway through picking up the edits on a new page the phone rang. I picked it up and the line went dead – bloody automated call centres. It had been happening a lot over the last two or three weeks. But then the phone had been busy all morning.

One of my boys was home with his new girlfriend for a few days and I wasn't ready to introduce him to Max. Not because of the BDSM aspect but because before I introduced them to any man I wanted to make sure the relationship was going somewhere before they met. I loved my kids far too much to introduce them to every new man I dated, and although I felt that Max was special, it was too soon.

It occurred to me, even as I was thinking that, that maybe that was what Max was worried about with his son; maybe that's why he hadn't suggested we meet up at his house. And me? Don't mind me: I'm the queen of double standards.

It wasn't that Max was unavailable. If we met on a Friday evening he'd send me an email as soon as he got back home and call me first thing on Saturday morning – early – while I was still in bed. The same if we met on a Saturday evening. It felt really good to be desired and wanted. Since we had first been in contact we had always talked about a lot more than BDSM – his job, my job, how the new book I was working on was coming along, my children, his children, his latest contract and the people he was working with. A film he would like to take me to see; the idea of having a weekend away together later in the year, even a holiday, which would give us a chance to explore what it meant to be together as Dom and sub for more than a few hours. Our relationship certainly felt like something special, but there was something in the background that I couldn't quite put my finger on. Give me a puzzle and I'm like a dog with a bone.

An email pinged into my inbox from Max. In the subject line it read: 'I keep thinking about you.'

I smiled. It seemed I wasn't alone in not being able to concentrate on work after all. Maybe I was wrong; maybe I should stop picking.

'You are my pleasure,' the email read. 'I want to feel your body under me; the heat of you, the smell and taste of you, fill my thoughts. I want you naked. I want to tie you down and beat you till you beg me for mercy. I want to take your mind and body to places that you can't begin to imagine. I want to breathe you in, I want you. I'm not sure if I can wait till Friday.'

Reading it and also knowing that none of it was an idle promise made my heart flutter. If it carried on like this it was going to be a long, long week.

'Slutty' is not a look I've paid much attention to over the years, so after going through my wardrobe and drawing a blank, I found myself trailing round the shops all week during my lunch hour, trying to find something that said 'fuck me' in an obvious way, but that I would be happy to run over in. I blame my mother. I can visualize the scene in A&E now: 'Ah, slutty,' they'd say as they cut away my fishnets and leopard-skin crop top. Lord only knows what they'd say when they discovered I hadn't got any knickers on.

Anyway, while I was running my finger along the rails of a rather nice dress shop in the high street and eyeing the price tags I wondered just how much I was actually prepared to pay for a dress that might well be ripped off me, given what Max had said when we'd been playing in the forest. That made me have a bit of a rethink.

'So,' said the lady in the charity shop, as she eyed the selection of things I'd piled up on the counter. 'A tart's party? That sounds like fun. We get a lot of vicars and tarts coming in here, don't we, Audrey?' she said to her companion.

I resisted the temptation to say anything. I'd already had her climbing into the shop window to retrieve a leopard-skin zipper-fronted micro dress with epaulettes and brass buttons. Fortunately it was too small for me, but it did make me wonder exactly what sort of clientele they were hoping to attract. To be fair, the ladies who volunteered in this particular charity shop have seen me through thick and thin over the years, their efforts including finding me a fabulous designer dress to go to a prize-giving in, so I shouldn't knock them or the service they give, and they'd really taken to the whole tart thing with zeal.

'This is one of your writing dos, is it?' said the lady, who had been assigned the task of calling out the prices, folding and packing.

'No, just a party,' I said casually, not quite meeting her eye, while trying to stop the pink feather boa sliding onto the floor. The consensus in the shop was that a quick shake in a bag with some flea powder, and then half an hour outside on the line and maybe a squirt of Febreze, and it would be as good as new.

The other lady, who was doing the 'putting the amount through the till' part of the transaction, looked down at the pile on the counter.

'Oh, you've got a nice lot there. Now let's see, what have we got then, Audrey?' she said to her friend, who obliged by reading out the labels.

'Stretchy black velour mini skirt £2.99; leopard-skin peeptoe sandals – look, they're brand new – £3.99, a bargain. I'll tell you what, out the back I think we've got a little velvet top, buttons down the front.' She mimed the shape over her sensible coral-pink twinset. 'It's a bit like a corset. Hang on, pet, I'll go and see if I can find it for you.'

You've got to love women like that.

She came back with a triumphant smile. 'There you go. Why don't you try it on? We'll put these on one side till you get back.'

The top was a bit tight and showed acres of what I'd like to imagine was voluptuous creamy white flesh – at least in subdued lighting – and was lightly boned and seamed, so that it gave me an impressive cleavage. To make the whole thing a little less revealing and a little less fleshy, the ladies found me a fabulous fitted, stretchy, black lace blouse on the 'Everything Must Go' bargain rail outside the shop doorway. Job done, I hurried home and put the whole lot in the washing machine.

So now all I needed to add were stockings, a suspender belt and a coat – and *voilà*, instant slut, and all for under twenty quid.

When I turned on my laptop there was another email waiting for me, flagged as urgent.

I would like you to remove all your body hair before Friday.

No need to ask who that was from.

I don't mind whether you wax or shave but I want you completely naked. I want to rub oil into the mound of your pussy, so it looks like ripe glistening dewy fruit, then turn you over and trickle warm oil all over your arse, and between the cheeks so I can slide my finger into you, feel the tightness of your backside, maybe fuck you there. You need to understand that there is no part

of your body that doesn't belong to me. No place that I
can't use for my pleasure. All mine, Sarah, all mine.

I stared at the words. I'd never experienced any of this,
never done it, never thought of doing it, but the words
were electrifying, and made the excitement and nervousness gather like storm clouds rolling in. I wondered how
the hell I was going to be able to wait until Friday and also
whether I really had the nerve to book into our local beauty
salon for a Hollywood ...

I didn't.

I was coming out of the shower on Friday evening when
the phone rang. For a moment I wondered if it might be
Max, but that seemed unlikely, unless he'd changed his
tactics. Up until now he usually let me stew in my own
juices on the day we were due to meet, with short texts
and emails to ensure that he wasn't far from my mind but
no phone calls; the day of the meeting, silence, which was
an interesting and very compelling tactic. The caller
display read 'number withheld', which made me think it
was probably Gabbie, ringing for an update. Her office
number always came up as withheld and she was the nosi-
est when it came to anything relationship-related.

She had already rung three times during the week and
I'd done my best to be chatty but basically evasive,
although that just made her all the more determined. One
thing about Gabbie was that when she was on to a scent
she was relentless, and she wanted to know all the ins and
outs of my relationship with Max.

I'd like to think she shared my concerns about him not spending the weekends with me but the bottom line was that she is just plain nosey, which is why I think we get on so well. As soon as I picked that phone up she would want to know what I'd got planned for the weekend with Max, right down to the last detail, and pick every bone clean. Any slip and obvious gap in the narrative and she would be on it like a terrier. Deciding what to tell her and what to keep to myself was a real work in progress.

'Hello,' I said brightly, while towelling my hair dry.

'Hello,' said a female voice. 'Is this Sarah?'

Something about the tone set off alarm bells in my head. 'Yes, it is,' I said cautiously. 'Who is this speaking?'

At which point whoever it was hung up.

It was odd and very slightly unsettling, and to be honest I wasn't sure if it was something or nothing. After all, people do ring, people do get cut off, and like everyone else I've had more than my fair share of cold calls from call centres. After a second or two I dropped the handset back in the cradle. If it was important they'd ring back, and anyway most of my thoughts were very definitely on other things.

My mother didn't raise a slut, so standing in front of the full-length bedroom mirror I did my very best to channel Bette Lynch or Bette Midler; or maybe, I thought, I should aim for what's her name in *Pretty Woman* (big ask), or Jerry Hall in the video with Bryan Ferry (nowhere near enough hair, lips or chutzpah). But none of it is easy when old-fashioned glamour is just not your style; take it too far and you find yourself slipping into pantomime dame territory.

So I went with marginally more lipstick, and a little extra eye shadow and mascara. Hooker-red lipstick made my skin look amazing, which was a revelation. I did momentarily toy with the idea of adding false eyelashes, but last time I wore them I ended up fishing one out of a man's prawn cocktail, so I decided on balance I was better off without. Hair a bit bouffant and off my face, like a young Kristin Scott Thomas (I wish), and I'd found a pair of big glitzy earrings in my jewellery box to add to the new look.

The clothes looked quite good, in a weird dressing-up kind of way, and the minute I slipped on the shoes it put me right into character (though I planned to take them in a bag – there was no way I could drive in them).

But the biggest change to how I felt was the whole shaving thing. Over the years I'd had my bikini line waxed and trimmed into a neat little arrangement, and I've had the odd tidy-up from time to time, but this was the first time I'd gone the whole hog and taken the lot off, and it felt odd – very odd. I looked in the mirror and slowly lifted my skirt. I felt exposed and vulnerable and more than naked. Rearranging my skirt, I picked up the long coat from the end of the bed, slipped it on, buttoned it up and hurried downstairs.

The coat covered me from neck to ankle because I didn't want my son seeing me dressed like a hooker. Not that I need have worried: he and his girlfriend were downstairs curled up on the sofa watching a DVD and didn't give me so much as a second look as I said goodbye and headed out towards the car.

As I drove to the hotel my imagination worked over-time on what Max had in store for me. Warm oil ... I replayed the contents of the email in my mind. The miles passed, the evening darkened. As I got closer and closer to my destination, among the anticipation I felt a growing tingle of excitement and quite a lot of nervousness; this feeling of edginess was part of the pleasure.

Finally I pulled into the car park and gave myself a few minutes to settle. I glanced at myself in the rear-view mirror, retouched my lipstick and put on the chandelier earrings, wondering if I looked ridiculous. I suppose that is one of the big fears, isn't it? That by dressing up and playing sexy and exploring your fantasies you set yourself up for ridicule. I took a breath. This was the game I had chosen to play.

I slipped off my sensible flats, trying to still my nerves, put the shoes in my bag and wriggled into the leopard-skin heels, locked the car and headed for reception. I'd been practising walking in the shoes all week, but they still made me feel as if I was playing dressing up with things from my mum's wardrobe. According to some fabulous camp guy on YouTube, the secret to walking in high heels is to walk slowly, concentrate on extending your leg and – and I've forgotten what the other things were, but whatever they were, they weren't working for me. I concentrated on climbing the steps, opening the door to the foyer and getting across to the desk without falling flat on my face – or worse.

The receptionist was young, wearing too much make-up and far too busy surreptitiously checking her hair in the reflection on the monitor to notice me hobbling across the vast expanse of plush dove-grey carpet. Just before I reached for the bell she looked up and painted on a smile.

'Good evening; my name's Chelsea; do have you a reservation?' she asked, all in one breath.

I nodded. Mr and Mrs Smith had seemed funny on the email; now it felt embarrassing. So only one way to go here: bluff confidence. If Chelsea had been older and brighter, I might have tried a joke, but instead I said, 'Yes, I have. I'm supposed to be meeting my husband here. Mr and Mrs Smith.' I applied a bit of extra cheeriness. She clicked the mouse and peered myopically at the words as they scrolled down the screen.

'I believe my husband left a parcel for me?' I added, glancing behind me just in case Max was somewhere watching.

'Oh, right,' she said. 'Mr Smith.' And, taking her eye off the booking screen, she started to rummage around under the desk. 'Here we are,' she said, smile broadening as she handed me an A5-sized padded envelope. 'Mrs Sarah Smith? That's it, isn't it?'

I nodded.

Chelsea beamed at me. 'Your husband told me it was a surprise.' She was animated now; obviously Max had made quite an impression. Her gaze moved back to the screen. 'Such a nice man. Right, here we are.' She activated a key card and handed it to me. 'Room one forty-two. That's in our annexe. First floor, room forty-two.' She pointed, and then glanced down at the envelope. 'Aren't you going to open it?'

Taken by surprise, I shook my head.

She looked genuinely disappointed. 'Will you tell me what was in it tomorrow?' she said. 'I'm on earlies.'

I smiled and nodded. 'If I see you,' I said. And I thought I was nosey.

Appeased, Chelsea pointed to the far side of the reception area. 'It's along the corridor – just follow it round. Forty-two is at this end on the ground floor, first door on the right. Have you got any luggage? Only it's a bit of a trek. I'll get the porter –'

'No, I'm fine. Thank you. I'll get my husband to come out and get it later,' I said hastily. Taking the envelope from her, I made my way across the foyer, trying hard to remember the things I'd read about high heels. Once I was out of sight of the reception desk I tore open the envelope and looked inside. Wrapped in pink tissue was a black silk mask trimmed with feathers and lace – the kind of thing you might wear to a masked ball, the only difference being that the eye holes were obscured with black velvet, so that the moment I put it on I would be unable to see. Nice touch. A typewritten note tucked inside said: 'Find room forty-two. Put your present on. Knock. Wait.'

I took a deep breath and headed down the corridor. Chelsea had been right. Forty-two was a long way from the main hotel, along a winding glazed corridor with views out over the garden and various lit water features. Have you ever had that dream where you walk for ever and never seem to get anywhere? It felt like that. I was going to be late after all, despite my careful planning. The corridor went on and on.

Finally I found the room, slipped the envelope into my bag, put on the mask, knocked and then waited. And waited. I could hear activity inside the room. I heard the door opening and I just hoped that it *was* the door to number forty-two and Max was inside waiting for me – that I hadn't done some weird numero-dyslexic thing and that some poor old bloke wasn't standing there in a towel thinking I was room service.

There was a moment then. A stillness. A settling.

I could hear music coming from inside and then some-one gently took my hands and led me into the room. I walked slowly, hesitantly, although it has to be said my fears about the shoes were fading fast. Someone took my handbag. I heard it drop down onto a surface a little way from where I was standing. My guide led me further into the room. I was nervous of tripping over something and reached out, trying to get my bearings. Firm hands lowered mine. I strained to pick out sounds and somehow get my bearings.

I wanted Max to say something, a welcome, some word of encouragement or greeting, but there was nothing: just the sound of something lush and classical with strings and flutes, and the thump, thump of my excited heartbeat pulsing in my ears.

On all the occasions I'd met Max before he had been wearing aftershave – nothing too brash or loud, something with sandalwood and musky low notes that had my mouth watering – but tonight there was nothing. No smell, no scent: just hands in the dark. Nimble fingers worked the buttons of my coat and slipped it off. I swallowed hard. I could have spoken. I could have taken the mask off, but I didn't. Instead, I revelled in the intensity and excitement. What had I been waiting for all my life if not for moments like this?

I could hear breathing – soft, regular, male, I was almost certain – and then I had a sudden moment of panic: what if this wasn't Max? My brain raced. Surely he wouldn't have set me up with someone else? That certainly hadn't featured on my wish list and certainly wasn't in the contract, was it? I started to tremble and lifted my hands towards my face, towards the mask. The same gentle hands dissuaded me.

Now those hands smoothed down over my shoulders, calming my panic, before tipping my chin this way and that as if examining me. Fingers worked through my hair and then traced a line down over my collarbones, before straying to the buttons of my blouse.

I shivered, but instead of undoing them his hands moved lower and pulled up my skirt over my hips, so that I was completely exposed. He stroked the mound of my sex, his palm cupping me, working up against the smooth, newly naked, shaved flesh. I wondered if he was checking up on whether I'd followed his instructions or not. Knowing fingers slid between the lips, opening me. I sighed with pleasure as he found my clitoris and began to stroke it gently, rhythmically.

God, I needed this; I had waited all week for this release. The little bud glowed white hot at his touch and

I moaned with pleasure. I might not know how to dress like a slut but my body had no problem acting like one. Within seconds I was moving in time with his fingers, feeling the pleasure building as he found a rhythm. I guessed it wouldn't take long. A finger slipped inside me and I began to drive myself onto it, seeking satisfaction. I should have known it wasn't going to happen that easily.

His fingers moved back up to my waist. And as I wailed in frustration, he caught hold of my shirt and ripped it open with one single violent movement, buttons careening off in all directions. I gasped in shock. He dragged it back off my shoulders, ripping and tearing, making me gasp before turning his attention to the corset top. One, two, three, the tiny buttons went the same way as those on my shirt. I shivered as the fabric gave way. He was moving. I could hear him. He grabbed hold of my wrists and crossed them behind my back.

Now I could feel the oil on his hands, feel him working it into my skin, pulling at my nipples, squeezing my breasts, finger and thumb pinching the tender areola, before his fingers eased up over my collarbones and neck, and then back down to my ribs, my shoulders, my arms. His touch was deft and hypnotic, fierce and then tender, every caress electrifying; I could feel myself getting more and more turned on. The oil, something heady and dark as wood smoke, made my head spin. I was floating on a sea of scent and sensation, and heard myself groan with pleasure as his attentions turned back to my breasts. He cupped their weight, thumbs circling my nipple.

It feels as though my nipples are wired to my clitoris. He touches, he sucks, he bites, and I am nothing but pleasure. Grabbing one breast, he starts to bind it with narrow cord. The cord bites into my flesh – to make it hold he needs it to be as tight as possible. The constriction makes me gasp as he binds and binds tighter, knotting it before starting on the other one. My nipples throb; where the cord nips my flesh it feels like a burn.

I heard the bells before I felt them, and instinctively – knowing what was coming – tried to step back, but not quickly enough. I was closer to the bed than I realized and, wrong footed, I almost stumbled. A hand steadied me, but before I had a chance to recover, his fingers caught hold of my breast. A split second later the little clamp bit down into my engorged, sensitized nipple. I whimpered and bit my lip, shivering with a heady mixture of excitement and pain.

Even so, as his hand took my other breast, I pulled away again. This time he caught hold of me by the shoulder, stopping me stepping away or falling back onto the bed. I could have called time, I could have easily stopped him, but I didn't; instead, I stood, trembling, waiting for the second clamp to bite. I tensed as his fingers caught hold of my nipple and pulled it taut. When the clamp bit, I let out a long throaty sob – it hurt. It really, really hurt. The bells echoed the sob. He opened my mouth and put the shaft of the crop between my teeth and pressed my jaws together.

I bit down.

I can hear his breathing, hear his arousal, and I am all feeling, consumed by the sensations. Something happens during these sessions: the pain, the pleasure, all the sensations build in layers, rendering me receptive and aroused, but oddly passive and totally absorbed in the way things feel. For me it is like an intense waking sleep, when every part of me feels connected and alive.

The sensations one after the other filled me up, overwhelming the receptors. I imagined what I looked like, how exposed, how vulnerable, yet a part of me was totally turned in on itself, feeling the rush.

Then he guided me up onto the bed – fleetingly I wondered if it was a four-poster – onto all fours, still with the crop in my mouth. He slipped off my shoes, rolling my skirt down, taking my stockings and suspenders with it. He worked with deft precision until I was naked except for my earrings and those tingling, tinkling clamps and ropes – every movement, every turn, every gasp was accompanied by the sound of the tiny bells. As my breasts tipped forward, the weight of them made them sway, down and forward, and the clamps tugged mercilessly. I whimpered as the pain flared and I wondered if this was something to do with my fantasy about Prince Charming – the one to whom I didn't need to speak. The one who knew everything I wanted and needed without me saying a word, although in my fantasy Prince Charming had never resorted to nipple clamps.

So now I was naked and he was free to rub the oil into my skin with two hands, over my back and thighs, my stomach, my legs, my feet, my breasts – there was nowhere his fingers didn't go, no places he didn't explore, even up over my face and into my hair. And all this time he didn't say a word, not one single solitary word. Then he unfastened the cords around my breasts and kneaded the flesh, making me gasp as the blood flowed back, making me writhe; then he turned me over, oily hands spreading my legs, working up inside my thighs, up over the swell of my hungry, desperate sex – this was a massage you would never believe. Then he stopped and I felt the oil start to warm, and then warm some more, until my whole body was tingling.

I gasped, letting the crop slip from my mouth.

The sensation built in intensity until it felt as if every inch of me was covered in sparklers, bright, hot twinkling lights; and as the tingling heat spread through me, he spread my legs wide and pressed his lips to my sex, hungrily, frantically, licking my clitoris, lapping, sucking, using his long tongue to lick me, till I was begging him to take me higher, to take me to the edge.

I was lost now; all thoughts of the little bells and the clamps that still rang in some other place in my head were subsumed in the glow from the oil and the sensations of pleasure his tongue was giving. As the pleasure began to build up, he pulled away and, desperate for more, I lifted my hips to chase his tongue – his magic, magic tongue – and as I did, something slapped sharply the arch of my pubic bone and the outer lips of my sex. The blow was sharp, stinging – it was narrow, like a ruler. I gasped, drew back, and he hit me again, not hard but in a tapping, tantalizing stream of blows, slowly building in intensity, harder now, now softer, faster, slower.

When I dropped back onto the bed so that he couldn't reach me, he dragged me over the edge of the bed, so that my hips and bum were over the edge, my feet flat on the floor, and then he hit me again, and again – tiny, stinging, tapping, flat strikes in a narrow area, hot, fast and amazing.

I was going crazy; I was so turned on that I thought I might faint. The warm oil, the building, throbbing, aching pulse in my clitoris, and the nipple clamps and that tap-tap-tapping rhythmic strike. I opened my legs wider, moving with the little blows, moving against them, drinking them in. The sensation grew and grew until it was overwhelming – then without warning, I was coming and I couldn't stop myself: it was there – it was there – and I could feel myself tumbling, tumbling and arching up to meet the next tap and the next as the pleasure flooded through me. It went on and on and on till I was a trembling wreck – I'd never felt anything like it. I also knew that he was there above me, watching me come – watching me lose control – and all for him, all because of him. He had done this to me, brought me to this place emotionally and physically, and at that moment I was completely his, a gasping, sweating, writhing animal, and I savoured every wild ragged sensation. There was no scrap of dignity, no false modesty left.

'You are such a slut,' he purred appreciatively.

And he was right. Hearing Max's voice made my heart leap. As I began to recover, he flipped me over back onto my belly, and grabbing me by the hips pulled me back up onto all fours.

I was breathless, undone, wanting nothing more than to curl up on the bed and gather the bits of me back together, but Max had other ideas. He poured more oil over my tailbone, letting it trickle down between the cheeks of my backside. I shivered: I knew what was coming.

His fingers parted my cheeks. I felt myself blushing, felt my embarrassment rising, as he explored the most secret parts of my body. He moved closer, one finger inside me, two fingers now – opening me up.

I am mortified, I am excited – I am truly not the me that I know.

Worse still, I feel my body responding to his touch. He steps away. I strain to pick out sounds that I recognize and then I'm sure – though I'm not sure how – that he is undressing. I hear him tear open a condom packet. I am so ready for him. He caresses and cups my sex, managing to rekindle the sensations that I thought were spent. His finger brushes my clitoris just as I feel his cock pressing between the engorged wet lips of my pussy, and more than anything I want him inside me.

I groan and instinctively flex my hips, tipping my pelvis up towards him – a primeval invitation. I am not disappointed. His cock is rock hard and slides home just as I feel his fingers stroking tightly the pucker of my backside, and a finger sliding slowly back into that most secret and tightest of places; and as I arch up onto his cock, I can feel him stroking his shaft through the soft membrane that divides one passage from another. I am ashamed by how much it turns me on.

I know then that I am all about his pleasure, not just mine. I feel like a toy that he has chosen from among many other possibilities, something there to delight him, something he wants and desires, something he wants to use; and something about that arouses and excites me. Pressing my face down into the bed, I lose myself in the moment, my intellect floating away on a river of feelings, letting our bodies find their natural rhythm.

Then, when I am absorbed by the way our bodies work as one, Max slips out and I know what he is going to do next. I gasp as he presses himself home; anal intercourse was never up there on my must-try list and I am stunned by the sensation. He moves slowly, letting me adjust. I am nervous. He is gentle, pushing forward slowly until my rogue body slowly opens for him; then his fingers slide around to brush my clitoris, reigniting the flame. The movements are more rhythmic now and I begin to move slowly, slowly, until we are back in time and I am no longer nervous, no longer holding back, and we start to move together, harder and faster, faster, harder, reaching for the end of the journey.

I feel him miss a beat, his breath is hard and hot on my skin, and I am coming and I can't hold back and he is coming and I am coming, and for an instant, one glorious instant, we are one – and I cry out in pleasure as the storm hits and rolls through us both, and we collapse down onto the bed, breathless, totally spent, exhausted.

And this time, as he slips out of me and slips off the condom, we curl up, back to belly, him with his arm around my waist, and I, closing my eyes, slide beneath the waves into a deep dreamless sleep.

* * *

I was disturbed much, much later by the sound of a door closing. It was very close by and I was instantly awake. For a moment I had no idea where I was or how long I'd been asleep. While I'd been asleep someone had taken off my mask and the nipple clamps. How could I not have noticed that? Someone had covered me – us – with a heavy chenille throw. *Us.* Which begged the question: if I was still curled up with Max, who was it who was leaving the room?

I rolled over. Max wasn't curled up around me. What I had taken to be him still snuggled up against my back was a bolster.

He'd dressed and showered and, damp hair brushed back off his face, he was standing by the sofa watching me. He was wearing jeans and a grey T-shirt; just seeing him made my mouth water. Desire is a strange thing.

'Who was that?' I said, bolt upright now, more meerkat than submissive, wrapping the throw around me.

'So you're awake, barely conscious and breaking the rules already?' said Max.

I didn't bother owning up; it was a fair cop. 'Was there someone else here?'

He raised his eyebrows, in a show of disapproval.

'Just now, when we were – were –' I wave my hands around, indicating the bed; words fail me. 'Was there someone else here watching us, Sir?' I tried.

He got to his feet and rattled a half-full tumbler of ice and alcohol in my direction. 'Would you like a drink? Something cold – or tea maybe?' He wasn't going to answer me: I could see that. Or at least I could see I wasn't going to get a straight answer. 'If you'd like to go and have a bath, I'll order us something from room service. Are you hungry?'

'I want to know who was in here, Sir,' I said, standing firm.

Max's expression hardened. 'No,' he said quietly. 'You don't. That's not the way it works. You don't need to know, Sarah. You need to have a bath.'

'It's a betrayal of trust if there was someone else here and you didn't say anything about it or warn me.'

Max appeared to consider what I'd said and then said, 'And what if I told you that there was someone else here? How would you feel?'

I stopped, feeling my colour rise. 'So was there?'

'I didn't say that. I asked you how you would feel.'

'I heard the door closing.'

Max nodded. 'What if I told you that there wasn't anyone else here?'

'I heard the door closing.'

'Then you've already made up your mind.' He paused, his eyes fixed on mine. 'Does it excite you to think that someone else was here watching us?'

I didn't know what to say. Yes, it did excite me, but in an abstract fantasy way – I didn't want to think too much about the reality of it – and at the same time no, because I'm not naturally an exhibitionist and there was a part of me that would feel shocked and betrayed that he hadn't asked me first. Whether there had been someone there or I had jumped to conclusions, it was obvious that Max wasn't going to put me out of my misery. Proving my point, he didn't say anything else; instead, he watched me as I mulled over my assumptions. Maybe I should have waited till I was more awake to have this conversation. He tipped his head towards me, his expression a question.

'I'm going to go and have a bath, Sir,' I said.

He nodded. 'Good choice. And no, there wasn't anyone else here. There is no way I would do that to you unless we had discussed it beforehand. Do you understand?'

'But the door?' I began.

'That was me; I needed to go and get something from the car. I didn't mean to wake you.'

As I stood up Max came over and took my hand, pulling me closer. 'Surely you know that I wouldn't betray your trust. You are amazing,' he said and before I knew what was happening he had leaned in closer still and was kissing me. It stopped me dead in my tracks. It was a real kiss, a proper boyfriend–girlfriend kiss. It felt good and made me grin – which made kissing tricky – and it made my heart do that whole thumpy-pitter-pattery thing. As he pulled away, Max's gaze caught mine. His eyes were dark and glittering, his expression intense and serious, and I wondered what he was thinking.

My grin held. 'I liked that. Can we do some more, Sir?' I teased. 'Or was that to stop me asking who was in the room?'

Max shook his head. 'No, not at all. I'm falling in love with you,' he said.

I stared at him, totally and utterly astonished. He sounded solemn, as if love was a burden. Maybe for him it was. Maybe this wasn't in his game plan. It certainly wasn't what I was expecting him to say. Finally his face cracked into a smile.

'You mean *real* love?' I said.

He laughed. 'Well, I hope so. What other sort is there?'

'Vanilla love.' Love that involved taking out the bins and waking up together, love based on easy familiarity and everyday things, not whatever this was.

He shook his head. 'I don't feel less because I'm a Dom; it's just different.'

'So where does that leave us?' I asked.

'It doesn't leave us anywhere. It's just the start, Sarah. The beginning – if you feel the same, that is.' He was grinning now.

I stared up at him. 'I do,' I said. 'You know I do. I was just worried in case there wasn't a place in what we're doing for real live love. And how can you love me when you've never seen me in my pyjamas or scraping cat sick off the carpet? You don't know me.'

Max shook his head. 'You think too much. Go and have a bath. I'll get us something to eat.'

As I settled back among the bubbles, I wondered if you really could combine a relationship based on BDSM with real life. It was a heady mix. The realist in me considered waking up every day with someone. Would he expect me to sleep on the floor for ever? Surely given time the magic would fade and become mundane? Could the dynamics survive familiarity? Could you seriously call someone Sir once you'd seen them slobbing out on the sofa in their underpants watching *Bargain Hunt*? And what about the physical side? Did it ever turn into cosy, comfort, snuggling-up sex or married sex?

Then Max came in carrying two glasses of champagne. His eyes working their way slowly over my body made me tingle with pleasure, and I wanted to kick myself. Here was I mentally hurrying through the good parts to the end, to the grey dull days of ordinary. It was early days yet – I was a fool to try to guess how this might develop over time. Far better to enjoy the ride than worry about the destination. No point wishing it away before it had even started.

Max sat on the side of the bath and picked up the soap and sponge. 'Supper in around forty minutes. Let me help you,' he purred. This time I didn't protest, want a question answered or come up with a smart answer.

Chapter Eighteen

'Why do you complain of your fate
when you could so easily change it?'
Marquis de Sade

I was driving home from the hotel in the wee small hours of the morning and my head was busy and my body sore, and I was sleepy and slightly spaced out from good sex and food overload and the unexpected possibility of love. Love. *Max said that he was falling in love with me.* Crazy. I found myself grinning like a lunatic as the dark miles rolled by.

It was the most horrible night; there were patches of fog in some places, rain in others, which made driving hard work. I couldn't remember a time in years that I had been up this late, and I couldn't work out why Max wouldn't let me stay all night with him. My eyes were sore and I'd done nothing but yawn for the last twenty miles.

Finally I pulled into a twenty-four-hour garage to buy a coffee to help me concentrate on the road and the foul weather and the poor visibility, instead of all the rest of the stuff clamouring for attention.

Love. *Really?*

It still sounded crazy. Did Max and I know each other well enough or long enough to be in love? When I met him I had had a feeling it was going to be something special, but love? Really?

And did I really want to be in love with a man whose idea of a good time involved flogging me? Could I spend the rest of my real life being tied up and caned?

Despite being tired, my brain kept replaying the last few hours. My nipples were bruised and tender, my body ached, I'd got my coat buttoned right up to the neck because the little corset top and the shirt I'd been wearing were both shredded and I was barelegged because my stockings were laddered and torn. I wanted nothing more than to be at home in my bed or back in the hotel with Max. I was just hoping the police didn't pull me over for anything.

While I was sitting on the forecourt, thinking about Max and whether there really was anyone else in the hotel room, I switched on my mobile phone.

The jingle fired up and had barely finished before the text alerts started rolling in, one after the other. There were six missed calls from an unknown number. I scrolled through to my voicemail. Six missed calls but no messages. I stared at the screen. I'd told my son where I was going (though not why) and I'm certain that if there had been a problem with my children or the house, or my parents, whoever it was who had rung would have left a message or rung the hotel. It's the kind of family we are – better to know and be prepared rather than blunder around in the dark.

I scrolled back through the missed texts. There were no phone numbers recorded for any of them, which seemed really odd.

Each of the calls was made at a few minutes after the hour, which made me wonder if it was some sort of automated call system – two minutes past eight o'clock, nine, ten, eleven, twelve. Odd. I switched the phone off and dropped it into my bag.

I finally arrived home as dawn was breaking. I was so tired that I could barely climb the stairs. Even so, the first thing I did was go upstairs into my office and check the phone. There were six 'number withheld' calls on there too, starting at 7.00 p.m. and then appearing on the hour every hour through until midnight.

In the morning, at a slightly more civilized hour, my son told me that there had been a whole series of hang-up calls, and in the end he'd just let the answering machine take them once he'd checked the caller display, as he was also convinced that it was some sort of automated dialler. Annoying but not unheard of, although if the same company was ringing my landline and then my mobile one call after the other that was definitely strange.

When I turned on my computer there was an email from Max waiting for me. One line: 'How easy is it for you to get away?'

Nothing else. No comment about the night before, no mention of love. Nothing.

'Why?' I wrote, and pressed 'send'.

'That'd be "Why, Sir, presumably?" came the reply seconds later.

One of these days I'd get it. 'Why, Sir?'

'I'm off to Paris next week. I've got to work but I wondered if you'd like to join me for a few days. Fly over on Tuesday and come back Sunday?'

The invitation stopped me in my tracks. I looked at the pile of editing on my desk. Maybe if I worked late and started early? To be honest, there was no contest.

'I'd love to, Sir,' I replied.

'Good. I'll arrange the flights and a taxi to get you to the airport. I miss you.'

I stared at the email a lot longer than was reasonable. Max missed me. I was still staring at it when the phone rang. The caller display said 'number withheld' and I was about to speak when a female voice said, 'Hi, is that Sarah?'

This time the voice sounded very familiar. 'Yes. Who is this?' I asked brusquely.

'It's Anita,' said the woman. 'We met at Georgina's party?' There was a question in her voice.

I didn't need any reminding who Anita was. I knew exactly who she was: the redhead who I'd got pegged as a troublemaker and to whom I'd taken an instant dislike – and if she had been the one making the no-message, hang-up phone calls I wouldn't be at all surprised. 'How did you get this number?' I asked coolly.

'That would be telling.' Her tone was teasing, inviting me to spar with her. I wasn't prepared to play.

'So how can I help you?'

'Oh meow. You shouldn't always judge a book by its cover, honey.' I wasn't sure what she was talking about. Did she mean I shouldn't judge her by her performance at

Georgina's? Or did she mean Max? And what was it in her tone that made me think that?

'I just wondered exactly how much you know about wonder boy?'

I felt my stomach lurch, but managed to resist the temptation to bite. I'd seen her at work at the party. 'I'm not sure what you mean,' I said, very evenly. 'I'm very sorry but I'm really busy this morning –'

'Wait,' said Anita, sounding less jokey. 'Don't hang up on me. What has Max told you about Abby?' She paused. 'Look, I know you think I'm a bitch, but believe it or not I'm trying to help you out here. The whole Anita brat thing is how I play, not who I am.'

'Really? I'm not sure what you're up to but –'

'Have you had any anonymous phone calls recently?'

That stopped me in my tracks.

'How do you know about that?'

'Because she did it to me too.'

'Who did?'

'Abby. It went on for weeks and weeks. And trust me it gets worse, much, much worse. I had to change my number in the end.'

'Abby?' I repeated. 'But why? Max told me that she left him for someone else.'

'She did. I think she thought the grass was greener. She ran off with some bloke she met on the internet. But I think she knew it was a mistake the minute she did it. Max is a good man – but I don't have to tell you that, do I? Now she's moved back to be near him, or didn't Max tell you that?'

'He did tell me.'

'Good. Did he also tell you she's just moved back in with him because she *accidentally* flooded the bathroom and now she can't live there till the electrics have been sorted out?'

I felt the breath being crushed out of my chest. 'Why are you doing this?' I hissed.

'Because I really like Max and I'm really pleased that he's finally found someone. The trouble with Abby is –' Anita paused as if weighing her words. 'Well, she is lovely but she is tricksy as hell and all "Oh poor me, look at how awful it all is." It broke his heart when Abby left him. I don't know if he told you, but we had a bit of a thing a few years back; it was something and nothing and we've stayed friends ever since. And when I saw him with you, I was so pleased he'd found someone nice, and I know he's got it bad.' She paused. 'I'm letting you know about Abby because Max is one of the good guys and he deserves to be happy. Abby drives him crazy. Anyway he said –'

'You've talked to him?'

Anita laughed. 'We talk a lot. Didn't he tell you? I work with him.'

I am beyond stunned. 'Are you serious?'

Anita was laughing now, although to be fair it didn't sound as though she was laughing at me; she just sounded genuinely surprised. 'He didn't tell you, did he? God, he is such a poker player, that man; always plays his cards close to his chest does Max. We don't work together all the time but –' she stopped. 'Look, all I'm saying is: watch yourself and don't let her get to you. I came to the conclusion that she doesn't want Max, not really, but she doesn't want to let anyone else have him either. She uses their daughter as a lever and all that "Help me, Max, I can't cope and I don't know what I'm going to do" bollocks is just a way of reeling him in,' said Anita, in a fair imitation of a high-pitched girlie voice.

'Wait,' I said, worried now that Anita was going to hang up. There were so many things I didn't know about Max and I wondered fleetingly if she might be the one to give me the answers, although I knew even before I began that it would be a deal with the devil. 'How did you get my number?'

'Max gave it to me,' Anita said breezily.

I couldn't believe that that was true. After a second she corrected herself. 'OK, so that's not strictly true; I stole it off his phone, actually. But I wanted you to know about Abby. Max deserves to be happy. I don't want her to come back and fuck his life up again.'

'Again?'

'Again,' Anita repeated darkly. I decided not to press her. I suspected it might not be the last time we'd speak.

'Thank you,' I said, and there was a part of me that meant it.

'Have you got a pen?' asked Anita. 'I thought you might like my phone number for when the shit hits the fan.'

'It might not.'

Anita laughed and this time I wasn't so sure that she wasn't laughing at me.

As I hung up I saw that while I'd been on the phone another email had arrived. It was from Max, with details of my flight to Paris.

Anita's phone call had left me feeling unsettled and confused, and with more questions than answers. I needed to talk to Max face to face, about Paris and about Anita, but most of all about Abby.

I knew he was good at compartmentalizing his life, and keeping secrets, although to be fair so far every time I had asked him anything Max had told me everything I wanted to know. Maybe it was just a case of finding the right questions and the right moment.

Chapter Nineteen

'Live today. Not yesterday. Not tomorrow. Just
today. Inhabit your moments. Don't rent them out
to tomorrow.'
Jerry Spinelli

Max sent a car to the airport for me. I'd never been to Paris
before. Sitting in the back, I watched as the landscape
unfurled under a bright blue Parisian morning sky. We
drove through the French countryside, past fields and
farms, and finally into urban sprawl as we hit the Paris
orbital, the Boulevard Périphérique, and then into the
heart of the city. The driver, when I told him I'd never
visited the city before, took me the scenic route so that I
could catch a glimpse of the Eiffel Tower and drive around
the Arc de Triomphe.

Max had booked us into a hotel tucked away in a narrow
backstreet that once upon a time, back in the mists of
time, had been the residence of some duke or other. The
driver carried my luggage inside while I registered and
then a uniformed porter showed me up to our room.

Max had taken a suite on the top floor with a terrace
that overlooked the cluttered, busy rooftops of old Paris.
A few feet from our terrace on the far side of the alley was

a tiny balcony set with a table and chairs, the little space festooned with flowers and vines, the shutters tightly closed against the heat of the day.

The walls of the buildings opposite were plastered and painted in faded soft ochres and umbers, the shutters dark brown, the paint peeling away to reveal the wood, now bleached silver by the unforgiving sun. I loved the faded beauty of it all and couldn't wait to explore.

The suite was something else entirely, and certainly wasn't faded. It was suffused with sunlight, muslin curtains blowing in the breeze, looking more like an advertisement for luxury living than any place I'd ever stayed in before. The colours were fabulous: old golds mixed with dark reds and peacock blues. There were flowers on the huge occasional table that sat between two sofas, and there was an envelope addressed to me, in Max's handwriting, propped up against the vase. Inside on a plain white card he'd written:

> Sorry I couldn't be there to meet you at the airport.
> If all goes well I'll be back by six. Until then, enjoy.
> Max

Below his message was written an address and a name. I glanced at the porter who was taking my case into the bedroom.

'Excuse me, do you know what this is?'

He took the card from me and then nodded. 'I know this place. You want me to get a taxi for you, madam?'

'What is it?' I asked.

He pulled a face, as if trying to find the words, and then smiled. 'Paradise,' he said, and then added, 'for women.'

He wasn't wrong. The address was for a spa, tucked away behind a parade of stylish shops. Max had booked me in for lunch, as well as a waxing, body massage, hair, nails, the whole shebang – more pampering in one long, long afternoon than I'd had in a lifetime. Sightseeing on hold, I spent the rest of the day there and practically floated back to the hotel in a cloud of perfume feeling as if there wasn't an inch of my body that hadn't been pampered, massaged and oiled.

When I got up to the suite, Max was sitting out on the terrace, sipping wine. Just seeing him there made my heart flutter. As I crossed the room, he looked up and his face broke into a broad smile, which mirrored my own. Still smiling, he held up a hand: he was on the phone. Standing up, heading my way, he spoke into the handset: 'Look, can we talk about this later? No, it's fine. I'll ring you tomorrow. I really have to go now.' And with that he slid the phone into his pocket. There was something about his tone, something warm, appeasing and soothing without trying to get caught up in the drama – and every last molecule of me knew, without being told, that he was talking to Abby.

'Sorry, I didn't mean to interrupt, Sir,' I said, part of me feeling as though I was intruding.

'You didn't,' he said. He looked me up and down, eyes alight with delight and desire.

'Work?' I pressed.

He smiled and shook his head. Did I push it a bit more; did I confront him with what I knew? No; instead, I grinned. I really was pleased to see him.

'Hello, Sir,' I said.

He laughed. 'Hello, Sarah. I'm so glad you're here. Hope you had a good day. Sorry I couldn't meet you at the airport. Put your hands behind your back and let me look at you.'

I wanted to embrace him, to say how pleased I was to be there with him, to ask him about the phone call and Abby and Anita, but instead I stood very still and waited like a good submissive, eyes down, while he inspected his possession.

'Are you feeling all right?' Max teased, as he walked around me slowly.

'I'm trying to behave myself, Sir,' I said.

'Good God!' He laughed. 'Really? I'm going to enjoy this. Come with me. I've got something for you.' He led me over towards the bed. On it was a large, flat, shiny cardboard box and alongside that two smaller rectangular ones. I'm not someone who is used to receiving presents, flashy or otherwise. I hesitated, feeling uncomfortable.

'Open them,' he said. 'Go on. I want you to wear them for dinner tonight.'

Inside the first, wrapped in tissue paper, was an expensive-looking black-and-white-print column dress with a black jacket.

'Oh, that is gorgeous, Sir,' I said, picking up the dress and holding it up against myself. It wasn't something I would have chosen, but there was no denying that the dress was elegant, beautifully cut and more stylish than anything I'd ever owned. As if reading my mind, Max said, 'When in Paris.'

In the boxes alongside it were red shoes and a matching handbag. The shoes – mercifully – though fabulous had kitten heels. 'They're beautiful,' I said. 'But –'

Max waved the words away. 'But nothing. It's for my pleasure. Try them on,' he said, settling down on the sofa with his wine, one arm slung casually along the back.

I folded the dress over my arm and made a move towards the bathroom. 'Here,' Max said, indicating a spot around three feet or so from where he was sitting. 'Put the dress down.'

I hesitated and then did as I was told. Slowly I unbuttoned my shirt. Try undressing in front of someone in broad daylight: it doesn't get any easier. He waited. Although I had gone to the spa in underwear, I had gone back to the hotel without any, guessing that he might be waiting for me. As my clothes slipped to the floor, I could feel Max's eyes working over my newly oiled, massaged and depilated body, taking in every curve, every line. His expression was impassive. At that moment I was entirely his. I might not always remember to call him Sir but my submission was never in any doubt.

When I was naked, Max beckoned me closer and indicated that I should kneel.

He unzips his fly and I creep forward to take his cock in my mouth. My lips close around him. He is hard in what seems like an instant and locks his fingers in my hair, pulling me down onto him, fucking me, pressing his cock deep into my mouth. Looking up, I see him lean back, throwing his head back, his expression ecstatic.

'Deeper,' he says.

I gag and struggle to breathe; he presses me down harder still. I struggle and whimper but he doesn't stop. I should never forget that however urbane, however generous and affable he is, he is a sexual sadist. I am gasping for breath.

When he is ready, when he has had as much as he wants or needs, he pushes me to one side and then face down onto the sofa, holding me down by my neck. I fight him, and when the pressure lets up, instinctively I crawl up onto the seat. He stands up and runs a hand over my back. My arms are folded under my face, my backside presented to him. His fingers explore me roughly and then he takes up a crop from the side table. How do I know? The sound: nothing sounds quite like it. I hear it cutting through the air. I flinch, but the first blow doesn't land as he teases me with the sound. I hear it again. This time the braided leather finds its mark: the tender, tender skin at the top of my thighs, just where the swelling of my buttocks begins. It cuts.

'I've missed you,' he says.

I cry out, struggling to stifle the sounds in the upholstery. I wish I could resolve the fight I have with the pain. Each time it hurts just as much as the first time, each time I hate it and I love it all at the same time, and each time it overwhelms me like water crashing over me, sweeping all control away. He hits me again. This time I shriek. He catches hold of my hair and jerks my head back.

'Open your mouth,' he says. I do as I am told and bite down onto the ball gag that he presses into my mouth and fastens tight. Then he hits me again. The tears roll down my cheeks as he gets into his stride, and I lose count of the strokes as the sensations drive away all rational thought. And then, finally, he stops. My breathing is little more than a series of ragged sobs as I feel his cock pressing between the lips of my sex, hard and hungry. He drives into me, making me cry out again as my body opens to him. As he presses deep into me, he leans forward and whispers, 'Touch yourself.'

I spread my knees and begin to move with him, my finger seeking out my clitoris as his hands settle onto my hips and he pulls me back onto him. He hunches over me, his fingers joining mine. The rhythm gets more frantic, more intense. I am gasping for breath now, crushed under his weight, whimpering and moaning around the ball gag. The noises seem to excite him more and he presses deeper still.

I feel the warm, raw heat building between us, the pleasure throbbing like a beacon low down in my belly, and then I am coming and cry out; Max is with me, his excitement feeds mine and mine his, in great white hot circles, and then we are done, falling forward onto the sofa, gasping and both laughing and spent.

* * *

We ate dinner by candlelight at a restaurant a few minutes' walk away from the hotel, a short stroll in the warm evening air. My new dress was a perfect fit without underwear, and the cheeks of my backside were striped with marks from the crop. As I sat down I had a sharp reminder of the pain that accompanied the pleasure. Max smiled as I winced.

The waiter handed Max the menu; he ordered for both of us.

We ate pan-fried scallops and steaks as soft as butter, and drank the red wine the waiter recommended. Max ordered dessert for me – a whisked concoction of cream and raspberries, topped with curls of dark chocolate – and cheese for himself. Words don't do the meal justice. The food was sublime, each mouthful an explosion of amazing flavours; the service was discreet and perfect, finding that fine line between attention and interference; and the wine was warm, dark and earthy. And while we ate, we talked and made plans for my sightseeing alone and the things we would have time to do together. He didn't need to tell me he was falling in love: I could see it in every gesture, every look, and I felt it too.

As we drank our coffee, he leaned across the table and said, 'Anita told me that she phoned you.'

I nodded. I'd been waiting for the right moment to bring Anita and Abby into the conversation but hadn't wanted to spoil the mood.

'She told me that you used to go out together,' I said.

'That's right, we did. It was only briefly, and a few years ago now. It was a bad time for both of us –'

'And Abby split you up?' I said, unable to stop myself.

'I'm not sure either of us were in it for the long term, but Abby certainly didn't help. Abby and I had not long broken up and she seemed to think that while it was OK for her to see someone else the same wasn't true for me. I'm not sure exactly what Anita told you, but it was messy and I don't think Anita ever forgave Abby.'

I nodded, not altogether sure what to say, but Max hadn't finished. 'I'm not sure if Anita mentioned that Abby is staying at my place at the moment with Ellie. She managed to flood the place she's just bought, and I said she could stay at mine until it's fixed. The builders are in this week and she should have moved back into her place by the time I get home.' He paused. 'I don't want you to think I'm hiding things from you.'

'But you are, Sir,' I said. 'You could have told me about Abby staying with you. I'm a grown-up. These things happen. It seems more suspicious if you don't say anything.'

He smiled and held up his hands in surrender. 'You're right, and I'm sorry.'

'I think Abby is phoning me,' I said.

Max didn't protest, instead he sighed and nodded. 'OK, leave it with me. I'll sort it out.' He paused. 'You are really important to me, Sarah. I don't mean to be secretive. All you ever have to do is ask and I'll always try and tell you what you want to know. Whatever it is.'

And I believed him, and while there were many things I wanted to ask, now didn't seem like the moment. I was just pleased that he had opened the door to talking more openly about what was going on in the rest of his life.

'Thank you, Sir,' I said.

We were the last to leave. As we walked back to the hotel, Max slipped his arm through mine and pulled me close. 'I'm so glad that you could come,' he said, and kissed me on the tip of the nose. As he pulled away and our eyes met, I felt that strange fluttery thing that happens and grinned like a loon. 'I wouldn't have missed it for the world,' I said, and he kissed me again, properly this time, and I felt myself melting into his arms.

I know about honeymoon periods and the sugar rush of first lust, but it was fabulous finally to spend real time together. Each night Max tied me to the bed and beat me before fucking me. There was no part of my body he didn't use, abuse or torment while I stifled my cries and tears into a pillow, and I loved every minute of it. And all the time the dynamic held: Max as the master, me as his submissive.

He had arranged for me to have a mattress on the floor alongside the huge bed that he slept in, which led to the hotel manager constantly asking me how my back was.

While at first I missed the intimacy of sharing a bed, each night when Max had done with me I would climb into my narrow single bed and sleep like a baby, which felt like sinking into a warm, velvety, dreamless black ocean. Each morning I was up before Max to run a bath and be ready for one of the staff to arrive with our breakfast, which we ate together out on the terrace. The rules were simple and unwavering, and oddly comforting.

While Max worked I took in the sights, and when he had finished work we explored together. The hotel was just a few minutes' walk from the Notre Dame Cathedral. There was so much to see in Paris, a few days really wasn't enough and I promised myself I would go back. I spent my time exploring the markets around Montmartre, the Basilica of Sacré Coeur, the Jardin des Tuileries and the Musée Rodin. Towards the end of the week Max took a couple of days off so we could go out together.

In the evening we ate in fabulous restaurants, caught up with each other's day, drank great wine, chatted and flirted, and generally enjoyed each other's company like any other couple.

Sex and submission permeated everything that we did. As we sat on the terrace in the evening after I'd showered and was sitting in my robe, he trickled hot wax from the candles over my breasts, stomach and shaved pussy, and then whipped the dried wax off with a riding crop, me gagged and desperately trying to be silent, to avoid attracting the attention of the couple in their sitting room in the little attic room opposite, watching TV.

He and I took a trip to the Louvre, me in a demure grey dress that he'd bought me, buttoned up to the neck, with flat shoes and devoid of make-up, the very epitome of humbled womanhood, but also braless, with no knickers and a narrow belt under my dress that circled my waist with a leather strap that went between my legs and was pulled tight, so that I was constantly aware of it pressing into my flesh. The Mona Lisa wasn't the only woman with an enigmatic smile.

As we admired the fabulous artwork, Max would stand behind me and rest a hand on my hip or buttock or thigh to remind me that I was naked under the dress – and, more importantly, naked for him; then he would catch hold of the belt between his finger and thumb and tug it gently to remind me it was there, and that my body was his.

We fucked on the terrace while the people across the alley ate their supper. He touched me in shop doorways under cover of darkness. I wore all-new rubber nipple clamps to dinner, without bells. The days were a blur of Paris's history, relentless sex, intimate secrets and pain. And I relished every last second of them. Every day seemed crammed full.

Max hired a car so that we could go a little further afield to the Palace of Versailles. As we explored the gardens around the palace, walking together in bright sunshine, chatting about lunch and what we planned to do in the afternoon, I began to think that maybe we *could* do this in the long term. The secret in the end to the way it worked was not about the kinky sex but about the dynamics between the Dom and his sub. The rules were absolutely clear: to make the BDSM relationship work I needed to trust Max to take care of me, which required complete submission of my will to his.

While I was with him I didn't find it that hard. It absolved me of responsibility and it was a breath of fresh air, a true moment of joy and release from my other world where I was responsible for everything. During the time I was with Max I didn't order a meal, pay a bill or make a decision. Each morning Max decided what I would wear. Over breakfast we talked about where we would go, what we would like to see – but once the decision was made I handed myself over to him completely.

And no, I didn't want this in every aspect of my life, and fortunately neither did Max. My independence had been hard won and I was not willing to hand it over to anyone for good, but for a few days it felt like a real holiday, and I felt wonderful, rested, loved and cared for in the most uncomplicated and basic of ways. I also knew that when I was away from Max he wanted me to be all the things that I am and more, but when I was with him I made the choice to give my power to him.

We talked about it as we explored the gardens.

'It's a question of trusting and learning to let go,' Max said.

I searched for a metaphor. 'Like ice skating?' I suggested.

'What happened when you went ice skating?'

'I fell flat on my bum and broke my wrist.'

Max laughed and handed me the bottle of water he'd been carrying. 'You maybe need a different metaphor.'

On the final evening before we were due to fly home Max took me back to the restaurant where we had eaten on our first evening. They could only offer us a booking for an early table, so we took it. The plan was to walk off supper along the banks of the Seine but I was cold, so Max suggested we should go back and pick up my jacket before we set off.

The streets and alleyways were bustling with people heading off to bars and restaurants, arm in arm, enjoying the evening and the ambience of the city. A man was playing a violin in one of the squares that we walked through and people were dancing. We definitely caught their mood.

Though Max had another few weeks' work in Paris, he was negotiating another contract in Rome and we were talking about spending more time together in both cities – doing all the tourist things, exploring the Coliseum and the ancient ruins of the Palatine, drinking in the little cafés together. I realized as we spoke that Max was factoring me into his future and I was doing the same with him and mine. As we got closer to the hotel, a stylish young man on a Vespa rattled by, and behind him, sitting side-saddle with her arm around his neck, was an exquisitely made-up woman, smoking a cigarette. When she saw us she blew a kiss.

As we got to the steps of the hotel I turned to Max. 'I've had the loveliest time, Sir. Thank you so much.'

Max grinned. 'Me too,' he said, lifting his hand to stroke my face.

'I won't be a minute. I'll just nip upstairs and get my jacket.'

'OK. I'm not going anywhere,' he said, glancing in my direction, but as I climbed the steps I realized that Max was no longer looking at me: instead, he was looking past me, through the glass doors into the hotel foyer. For an instant he froze, a look of disbelief on his face. I turned to follow his gaze.

Sitting by the reception desk was a small blonde woman. She was sitting right on the edge of her seat, as if she was waiting for something or someone, all coiled and ready to spring to her feet at any second. She had a coat folded across her knees and an overnight bag at her feet. Sitting alongside her was a little girl, who was holding the handle of a Kitty Pink pull-along suitcase.

The instant the little girl spotted Max her whole face lit up and she jumped to her feet. You didn't have to be any kind of lip reader to see what she was saying. 'Daddy, Daddy,' she called, and she was across the foyer before Max was even halfway up the steps. I stepped aside as he hurried past me. She struggled to open the heavy glass door, and Max was instantly there, opening it, swooping her up in his arms and hugging her tightly, masking his surprise. If he was annoyed or angry or perturbed by the two of them showing up, he didn't show Ellie. And me? I was dead in the water, watching them.

'Hello, sweetheart,' Max said, holding Ellie close, before turning his attention to Abby. I followed on behind, feeling like an extra in a soap opera.

'What are you doing here?' he asked Abby, as Ellie climbed him like a tree. His tone was very calm and measured. It felt to me like they had been here before. It was Ellie, not Abby, who answered: 'Mummy said that we could come and see where you were working and go out for ice cream with you.' She was obviously dog-tired, and slipping her arms around his neck she curled into him, slipped her thumb into her mouth and settled her head on his shoulder. 'I'm hungry, Daddy.'

Max lifted a hand to smooth her hair. The gesture, so tender, brought tears to my eyes. I felt as though I had no place there watching them.

'You wouldn't take my calls,' Abby said, as if that explained everything. 'I didn't know what else to do.'

Behind the desk the receptionist was listening from a discreet distance. I've no doubt he'd heard it all before, but I recognized a cocked ear when I saw one. I went over to him to collect the room key, making sure I didn't catch Abby's eye. He handed it to me without a word. I thanked him and made my way towards the stairs. I didn't hurry. I didn't want Abby to think I was running away or that I was afraid of her.

Whatever was going on between Abby and Max, I'd got no plans to jump into the middle of it. They needed to sort it out for themselves. I'm not good with scenes, and despite the fact that I'm extremely nosey, however curious I was about Abby – and I was – although there was a part of me that was horribly tempted to hang about on the stairs and eavesdrop discreetly, I planned to go upstairs and let them get on with it.

'Where are you staying?' I heard Max ask, and braced myself for what I guessed was going to be the answer.

'I don't know,' Abby said. 'I didn't think. I just had to talk to you, Max.' Abby sounded fragile, and I decided cynically that from where I was standing it looked like a well-honed act. She was tiny – maybe five feet one or two, with big brown eyes and short hair that framed elfin features. She could have been drawn by Disney. I could easily see why Max would be attracted to her. She looked over in my direction. Her expression was triumphant.

'You don't know who I am, do you?' she said in a crisp, clear voice. 'Did Max tell you about me?' Although she said it evenly, there was a hint of something altogether more hysterical just below the surface. I didn't meet her eye and carried on walking towards the stairs. Her voice followed me. 'I said, "Do you know who I am?" Do you?'

Max started to quieten her but Abby was having none of it.

I turned slowly and nodded. 'Yes, I do, Abby, and I'm sure that whatever it is you have to discuss with Max it would be a lot easier if I wasn't here.' As I spoke I could feel my heart thumping like a drum in my chest.

She glared at me. 'Oh, that's it, run away,' she said. 'He loves me, you know.'

Max gently took hold of her arm, but looked up at me, and nodded in gratitude.

It didn't take a genius to see that Abby was slowly coming apart. I couldn't imagine how desperate she must have been to fly out to Paris with Ellie.

When I didn't respond, her lip curled. 'You're not the first, you know. Did he tell you that we're living together again now? Did he? Max can't live without me. He invited me back. I've told him we ought to have another baby. It would be good for Ellie to have a baby brother or sister.'

I glanced at Ellie. She was still on Max's hip, her head on his shoulder; she had her thumb in her mouth and her eyes were closed. She was the only one I felt any real sympathy for.

It was almost midnight by the time Max finally came back upstairs to our room. I'd been thinking a lot about what I was going to say to him, imagining what he might say to me, trying to second-guess the conversation we might have, but as it was we said nothing. As he opened the door I saw everything I needed to know on his face.

He took me in his arms and hugged me and held me close against his chest. I could feel his heart beating against my cheek. He didn't need to say anything. Not a word.

Finally, Max sighed and pulled away. He poured us both a glass of wine and carried the glasses out onto the terrace.

'I've booked Abby into a hotel. About five minutes from here. The guy on reception sorted it out and got them a taxi. Ellie's exhausted.'

I nodded.

We sat down at the table, our knees touching.

'I'm sorry. I really had no idea that she would show up here, Sarah. She said she was moving back to be near her mum and dad, and I thought it would be all right, and then she flooded the house.'

I didn't say anything. What was there to say?

'She's not well.' Max rolled the bowl of the glass around between his fingers. 'I didn't invite her to move in with me. She just turned up with Ellie. She's got lots of problems.' He paused. 'She needs help. She wants me to take her back.' He looked grey with tiredness and heavy-eyed.

I nodded. 'And what about you: what do you want?' I asked quietly. On the arm of the chair I was sitting on I could see a splash of the wax Max had used when we had been playing outside earlier in the week.

He ran his fingers back through his hair. 'You know what I want, but there's Ellie to think about. I really worry about her.' He paused, 'At the moment they both need me.'

I nodded. I could see the dilemma and didn't envy him the place in which he found himself. Of course it wasn't the answer I had been hoping for, but it wasn't unexpected and it helped me come to a decision.

That night, for the first time, we slept together, curled up in each other's arms.

I was up early and started to pack. By the time Max was awake I had showered and dressed and was ready to leave. Max looked vulnerable, dark-eyed and tired, and in the half-light of the bedroom I realized just how much I could love him if I had the chance.

'What are you doing?' he asked.

'Going home,' I said, without a hint of side.

'Your flight's not until lunchtime.'

'I know, but I'd rather wait at the airport, and you need to talk to Abby. I'm sure she'll be expecting you,' I said and then paused. 'There are lots of things that you need to sort out.'

'Are you leaving me?'

I struggled not to cry. 'No, I'm falling in love with you, Max, you know that – and that's the problem: I don't think you're ready. I saw the way you looked at Abby last night. You're not over her, and you're right: she's not well and she needs help. You love your little girl, and who can blame you? I can see that at the moment they both need you.'

'Are you asking me to choose?'

I shook my head. 'No, of course I'm not, but I've come too far on my own to settle for a compromise. I want to be with someone who wants to be with me.'

'But I do,' he said.

I understood. He was saying the right things and I knew that some big part of him meant what he said, but I could also see the conflict in his face. 'I know you do, but you need to sort this out with Abby,' I said gently.

Max nodded. I could sense the relief.

I bent down to kiss him goodbye and then I held out my hand. His face held a question. I touched the necklace he had given me. Very slowly he took the key ring from the bedside table, unfastened the key to the padlock and gave it to me. I smiled, picked up my suitcase and left.

I'd never done anything like that before – not walked out on something that I really wanted and believed was love and had a future; but I could see with blinding clarity the mess I'd be heading into if this carried on, and for once I was wise enough not to be pulled in. If Max truly wanted me, then he needed to sort his life out first. Would I wait? The truth was that at that moment I wasn't sure. My instinct was that Abby would feature in his life for a long time to come and I wasn't sure I wanted to put my life on hold.

Does that make me heartless and unsupportive? I don't know. One of the things I'd learned about being on my own was that, when it came right down to it, the only person who could truly take the best care of me was me – and if Max was meant to come to me he would.

I cried all the way to the airport. As I sat in the departure lounge there was a big, big part of me that hoped Max would come after me, beg me to stay, promise me that he would love me for ever, but another more pragmatic part knew that he and Abby were probably walking around Paris together, eating ice cream, hand in hand with Ellie.

Chapter Twenty

'What is broken is broken – and I'd rather
remember it as it was at its best than mend it and
see the broken places as long as I lived.'
Margaret Mitchell

When I arrived home there was a message on the answering machine from Max. Two words: 'Call me.'

I listened to it several times, listened to his beautiful voice, listened to the tone, trying to squeeze every nuance, every last clue from those two words. Then I deleted it and rang Gabbie.

'Gabbie?'

'Hi, Sarah. How was Paris?' she said, all bright and breezy.

I didn't know what to say; she sounded so happy, so curious, and I was in bits. Instead of words, all that came out was a strange sob. Of all the ways I had imagined my relationship with Max developing it has to be said that this wasn't one of them.

'What's happened?'

I took a deep breath. 'I've been very sensible and very grown up and now I feel like shit,' I said. Then I burst into tears.

'I'm on my way,' Gabbie said.

She brought tequila.

Gabbie owns a tiny one-bedroom cottage in a row of other tiny cottages down on the coast – not the glamorous coast but the countrified coast – in an unfashionable village flanked by bigger flashier places, and for some reason much favoured by lesbian lady hikers. After a night of tequila and much talking, I drove down there with my laptop, my editing, the dog, comfort food, a car boot full of logs and my walking boots.

There's no Wi-Fi, no broadband, and the only place you can get three bars of a mobile signal in the whole village is by the jukebox in the pub, which was where the dog and I went for lunch most days.

I sent Max an email before I left:

Dear Max

I hope you are OK. I have had a fabulous, wonderful, blissful time with you. Thank you for being all the things I hoped you would be and more besides.

I truly hope that you and Abby can find a way to sort things out between you. The truth is I don't want to get caught in the crossfire.

You asked me if I wanted you to choose, but you shouldn't need to. If you really wanted to be with me the question wouldn't have arisen. I could see you were torn and that you still have feelings for Abby, and I can perfectly understand that. I'm not normally this clear-sighted, Max, but I can't afford to fall in love with someone who isn't completely free to love me back. And, even though you may want to, I know you're not free. I wish you well and

My fingers hesitated over the keys. I backspaced and wrote:

> I wish you all the good things you deserve. You are a lovely guy and I had hoped – well, you know, I'm going to miss you.
> With kind regards and much love,
> Sarah

I cried some more, and then I pressed 'send' before I could change my mind, went outside and loaded the dog into the car.

Cold turkey, warm fires, wall-to-wall work and brisk windy morning beach walks with the dog cleared my head a treat. I'm a great believer in 'what is yours comes to you', and if I was meant to be with Max then I would be.

And even though it was one of the most painful things I've ever done, I knew that I had done the right thing – or at least I knew some of the time. Some of the time I cried, and some of the time I took my mobile to the pub and dialled Max's number but didn't press 'ring'. I tried to come up with ways we could be together. I composed endless emails to him in my head, but the truth is that I didn't know what it was I wanted to say. Or maybe there were just too many things to say.

Edits done, book finished, I drove home a fortnight later, nearly a stone lighter from all the thinking, the walking and the heartache and the way those things made everything I ate taste like wet cardboard and chopped hay. Knowing I was doing the right thing didn't make it the easy thing.

When I got home, the dog sloped straight upstairs to my office and hopped into his basket and I woke my Mac up and opened up my email.

There was one from Max. It was very simple.

It said that he loved me and that his heart hurt when he thought about me, but at the moment Abby and Ellie needed him, and for now that was where his focus had to be. He hoped that we would be able to stay friends. And who knew what the future might hold?

There was more, a lot more, but it makes me cry to write it down. I think we both believed that we had found something incredible and special and were both very sad when we decided to walk away from it.

When I closed the email down I took the key from my handbag and unlocked Max's necklace, which I had worn every single day since Georgina's party, put it back into its box and put it away in my desk drawer.

And yes, even though we had agreed it was over, there was still a big part of me that hoped he would email, or ring or just turn up and say he had made a mistake – but with each passing week that hope slowly faded.

I started to work on the outline for my new book, took on some more teaching, started writing for magazines, did the garden, walked the dog. Work, work, work – nothing like it for taking your mind off an aching heart. I also wasn't eating much, so the weight was staying off. The heartbreak diet – maybe there really was a book in that: whimper yourself slim.

Early one evening a few months later the phone rang. It said 'number withheld' and I wondered if it might be Gabbie – I'd left her a message suggesting that it was high time that we had a girls' night in or out and I promised not to cry, but instead a male voice said, 'Hi, is that Sarah?'

I hesitated. 'Yes, it is. Who's speaking?'

'I don't know if you remember me. My name's Alex. We spoke a while back about your ad.'

'We did? What ad?'

'Oh, I'm sorry. Maybe I've got the wrong number.' He sounded slightly flummoxed. 'It was quite a while ago now. You were looking for a Dom.'

'And we spoke?' I said. I had taken the ad down when I started seeing Max regularly and I hadn't felt anywhere near ready to put it back on the site.

'Only briefly,' Alex said. 'You were just off to meet someone and said you didn't think it was fair to talk to me until you'd met him. Anyway, I was going through my inbox just now, saw your name and thought I'd give you a ring.' He laughed. 'Nothing ventured ...'

I pulled up my email file and put 'Alex' into the search panel.

'To be perfectly honest I'm not looking at the moment,' I said, eyes working down the list of names. His wasn't there, although after meeting Max I had deleted other contenders.

'Bad experience?' asked Alex. It was interesting that he didn't assume I was living happily ever after in nipple clamps and leg irons.

'No, not at all. Just –' I felt around for the right word.

'Complicated?'

'Kind of,' I said, wondering why I didn't just hang up.

'Me too. I was chatting to this woman online for a couple of months, Annabel. She sounded perfect. Anyway we arranged to meet, and it turned out she was a bloke, Archie – fourteen stone, five feet two, buck teeth and –'

'You're joking.'

Alex laughed. 'Yes, actually I am, but not completely. We started to see each other and I discovered that she was married and just looking for a bit of kinky fun on the side – not really my style and not what I'm looking for. I was wondering: how about we meet up for lunch and swap horror stories?'

Now it was my turn to laugh. 'That's a bit of a leap.'

'True, but I'm not a stalker or a loony. I've been divorced four years and I've spent a lifetime thinking about this. I'm a newbie too, so it would be good to talk to someone who is looking for the same thing that I am.'

'Which is what?'

'True love, world peace and to be able to play the guitar like Ry Cooder?'

'I'm not sure about world peace.'

'OK. So tell me some more about you,' Alex said.

'Haven't we already done this?' I asked.

'Probably, but it was a long time ago now. I've probably forgotten all the interesting bits. Let's do it again. Do you like fish?'

'What?'

'I have a friend who runs a great little seafood restaurant on the coast. I was thinking we could maybe meet there.'

The last thing I needed now was another man in my life. I'd been thinking that maybe it was time to kick back, take time out, give up men and get some cats. 'I'm not sure –' I began.

Alex laughed. 'No, me neither. How about we just give it a go? I promise not to be weird.'

I hesitated. Oh, what the hell. 'OK,' I said, 'but the first hint of weirdness and I'm out of there.'

'Good call,' said Alex. 'When do you fancy meeting up? Are you free this weekend?'

I went through the motions of opening my diary and flicking through the pages, giving myself time to think, wondering whether I really was ready to start over. Did I really want a relationship based on BDSM? Did I want to play again? The truthful answer was yes and unless I planned to spend the rest of my life alone there was no way I was going to find a BDSM or any other kind of relationship running scared, hiding away in my office.

'Sunday?' I suggested, in a tone that I hope implied I might just be able to squeeze him in to my hectic social calendar.

'Sunday's fine,' he said. 'Say one o'clock?'

'OK.'

'I've still got your email address here. I'll book a table and I'll email you a map.'

'OK.'

He laughed. 'So far, so good. You want me to hang up now?' he asked.

'Maybe, unless you've got something interesting to say, or are you saving that for Sunday?'

'Oh, very sharp,' he said, aping a wince. 'I'll go.'

'Alex, wait,' I said hastily.

'What is it?' he said.

'Can you send me your profile again? I don't think I kept it.'

'I certainly can.' And this time the laughter was even louder.

'Good job I'm thick-skinned.'

Epilogue

I need to say something about the events, people and places in this book. This is not a how-to manual. I'm certainly not advocating BDSM as a lifestyle choice for everyone, or in fact anyone who is not already drawn to it – and believe me, I suspect if you are drawn to it then you already know who you are, even if you've done nothing about it.

This book is about my own personal experiences and they are far from a definitive guide. I've played in one tiny corner of what is a vast empire of alternative encounters. Yes, I took some risks – quite a lot of risks – but *they were all my choice*. I was not coerced or bullied into taking them. I'm not a doormat or a victim and I'm certainly not advocating anyone else does what I did. In fact, as your good friend I'd probably try to talk you out of going through with some of them or tell you off afterwards for being stupid – which was exactly what my good friends did with me when I finally let the cat out of the bag and let them know what I was up to.

I've also had some fabulous times with wonderful people, whose privacy and lifestyle I respect and value, and who I feel privileged to have met. To protect them and their lifestyle choices I've changed their names, their appearance and their age. And while everything in the book is based on my life, I've blurred the edges and the conversations here are, obviously, purely my recollection of them – I find it hard to take notes when I'm tied up. The places where and the times when the events took place have been changed. Those who shared their secrets, their passions and their bodies with me are, I hope, still there in essence, but not in sufficient detail to reveal their identities.

I'd also like to make it crystal clear that what I enjoyed from exploring and living the lifestyle was not abuse; nor should it be confused with bullying, casual brutality, cruelty to women or men, or domestic violence.

One of the sweetest and most telling moments to illustrate this was finding myself tied up on a huge wooden frame, naked except for a sparkly mask, a dog collar and a pair of fabulous strappy sandals. As my would-be tormentor stepped closer to ensure I was tightly bound, he trod on my toes and was desperately apologetic. 'God, I'm so sorry,' he said, bending down to see if he had done any damage and rub my toes better. 'I didn't mean to hurt you. Are you OK?' This from a man who two minutes later would be using a riding crop to raise some extremely spectacular welts across my backside.

Everything that happened to me and to those people I encountered was consensual and safe, in the sense that my health, my mental well-being and the health and well-being of those involved were a top priority, and I had a great time and lots of fun. I wish I could say the same about some of the 'normal' relationships that I've been involved in over the years.

Am I glad I met Max? Absolutely. As a first Dom I can't think of a better person to have shown me the ropes (literally) or to have guided me through the basics of BDSM in a safe, sane and consensual way. I had a blast. But being with Max also made me think about the things I really wanted in a relationship. After we broke up I realized that I wanted someone who could enjoy BDSM but enjoy vanilla too, who could tie me up and cuddle me afterwards, for whom good vanilla sex was as important and as fulfilling as tying me to a tree and whipping me till I wept.

Did I find him? Yes, I did, and, reader, I married him and live the lifestyle of what passes for ordinary in my neck of the woods. There are days when he ties me to the bed and others when we curl up in it and read, snuggled up and cosy. Sometimes I wear a leather corset and fishnets, but most often I wear gardening gloves and jeans, and BDSM is just another part of the rich pattern of our lives together, an interesting and exciting aspect of our sex lives, but not all of it.

For me my journey into BDSM was, and continues to be, a final and happy acceptance of a part of my nature.